When a Child Has Diabetes

Denis Daneman, MB, BCh, FRCPC
Marcia Frank, RN, MHSc, CDE
Kusiel Perlman, MD, FRCPC

FIREFLY BOOKS

A FIREFLY BOOK

Cataloging in Publication Data

Daneman, Denis
    When a child has diabetes

(Your personal health series)
Includes index.
ISBN 1-55209-331-X

1. Diabetes in children—Popular works. I. Frank, Marcia.
II. Perlman, Kusiel. III. Title. IV. Series.

RJ420.D5D36 1999   616.92'462   C98-932594-6

The statements and opinions expressed herein are those of the authors, and are not intended to be used as a substitute for consultation with your physician. All matters pertaining to your health should be directed to a healthcare professional.

Published in Canada in 1999 by Key Porter Books Limited, in conjunction with the Canadian Medical Association.

Published in the United States in 1999
by Firefly Books (U.S.) Inc.
P.O. Box 1338, Ellicott Station
Buffalo, New York, USA
14205

Diagrams: Lianne Friesen
Electronic formatting: Heidy Lawrance Associates

Printed and bound in Canada
99 00 01 02   6 5 4 3 2 1

*For those whose lives are touched by diabetes,
and those with diabetes whose lives have touched us.*

Canadian Medical Association Advisory Committee

Daniel L. Metzger MD FAAP FRCPC
Endocrinology and Diabetes Unit
British Columbia's Children's Hospital
Vancouver, BC

Sarah Muirhead MD FRCPC
Pediatric Endocrinologist
Children's Hospital of Eastern Ontario
Ottawa, ON

Danièle Pacaud MD FRCPC
Pediatric Endocrinologist
Alberta Children's Hospital
Assistant Professor
University of Calgary
Calgary, AB

Contents

Acknowledgments / vii

Foreword / ix

Introduction / xi

Chapter One: Overview / 1

Chapter Two: Striking a Balance / 22

Chapter Three: All about Insulin / 33

Chapter Four: Making Meals Work / 53

Chapter Five: Balancing Blood Sugar / 72

Chapter Six: Handling Highs and Lows / 96

Chapter Seven: Adjusting to Diabetes / 117

Chapter Eight: Growth and Development / 138

Chapter Nine: Putting Complications in Perspective / 163

Chapter Ten: Setting the Stage for a Healthy Future / 179

Chapter Eleven: The Future of Diabetes / 190

Glossary / 201

Further Resources / 204

Index / 210

Acknowledgments

We would like to acknowledge a number of individuals who have made direct and important contributions to this book. Three current or recent members of our diabetes team at The Hospital for Sick Children provided their expertise in co-authoring specific chapters: Margo Small, MSW, the team's social worker, made major contributions to Chapter Seven and Chapter Eight; Cheryl Miles, RD, and Marilyn Fry, RD, CDE, until recently the dietitians on the team, brought their experience and wisdom to Chapter Four. Janice Biehn has provided enormous writing and editorial support; without her constant encouragement the book might never have seen the light of day.

Other members of the diabetes team have provided ongoing support, and have reviewed the information to ensure accuracy and comprehensiveness. They include our diabetes nursing colleagues, Ana Artiles-Sisk, RN, CDE, Monica Bulmer, RN, CDE, and Janet Ruston, RN, CDE; and our fellow pediatric endocrinologists, Dr. Étienne Sochett and Dr. Diane Wherrett. We all owe a large debt of gratitude to Dr. Robert Ehrlich, the originator of the interdisciplinary diabetes team at The Hospital for Sick Children, who encouraged and supported all three of us as we started our careers in diabetes care.

Denis Daneman, MB, BCh, FRCPC
Marcia Frank, RN, MHSc, CDE
Kusiel Perlman, MD, FRCPC

Foreword

The discovery of insulin by Frederick Banting and Charles Best, at the University of Toronto in 1921, suddenly and dramatically changed the outlook for people with Type 1 diabetes. No longer was it a fatal disease, and no longer did health care professionals need to watch helplessly as children succumbed. Now there was treatment. The Hospital for Sick Children in Toronto quickly made a commitment to the care of children and adolescents with diabetes, a tradition that continues today. One of the first physicians to become involved in both diabetes care and research was Dr. Laurie Chute, followed by such eminent clinicians as Dr. Harry Bain and Dr. Robert Ehrlich.

In the 1960s it became evident that diabetes care and education were too complex to be handled in the traditional medical model—that is, through occasional visits to the doctor by the child or teen and his or her family. Rather, what was needed was an interdisciplinary health care team consisting of physicians, nurses, dietitians and behavioral specialists, all bringing their unique training and expertise to bear on the care of this complex condition. The diabetes team was the first of the interdisciplinary teams now standard in many areas of health care.

Since most diabetes care occurs in the home, at school or elsewhere outside the hospital or doctor's office, it has also become apparent that the care of children and teens with diabetes requires a family-centered approach: both the child or teen and the family are intimately involved in decisions that affect not only the diabetes, but all aspects of their lives.

This book is intended primarily for those involved in the care of children and teens with diabetes: parents, other family members, teachers and other school personnel, sports coaches, camp counselors and others, not forgetting the children and teens themselves. It is essential that those affected know as much as possible about the disorder. While we do not intend to present the last word on every subject, we hope you will find this a useful first step in learning about diabetes and its management, and a comforting reference when things seem not to be going quite according to plan.

Where does our information come from? We have all learned from our training, our mentors, our day-to-day work and, most particularly, from the children, teens and families whose experiences with diabetes constantly yield new information, new approaches and new coping strategies.

There are a few important caveats to remember as you read this book. First, different diabetes health care teams have different approaches to some or all of the aspects of diabetes care we deal with here. If you are confused by something we have written, or it conflicts with the approach of your health care providers, discuss it with them. Most often you will find that what we have provided is a variation, rather than a radically different approach.

Secondly, this book was written in 1998—things change! We can all hope that biomedical research will advance our understanding of many aspects of diabetes care in the foreseeable future. So expect an evolution in our thinking in years to come.

Finally, not everything works for everybody. If something doesn't seem applicable to you or your child, discuss it with your team. Once you have a good understanding of the condition, work with your team to do some further experimentation. Try things out and see how successful they are. If they work well, tell us about them—we're always ready to learn.

We present this work in the proud tradition of excellence in diabetes care, education and research that has been the trademark of The Hospital for Sick Children for more than 75 years. If in some small way it lessens the burden of diabetes management for our readers, we will have fulfilled our mission.

Introduction

Heather is nine and she's a livewire. A tall, thin child with straight blonde hair and bangs, she's bright and bold and independent. Drama is her forte and she sings and travels with a children's opera chorus. For Heather, each new experience is an adventure; she refuses to let diabetes change her life.

Tommy is a charming, cherubic child of two and a half. He spends hours pretending he's a firefighter, gathering his siblings and playmates into fire-fighting squads. Tommy has diabetes and these days he would much rather "cook" in his play fire station than eat real food. His unpredictable eating makes it harder to manage his diabetes safely.

Sonia is in the tenth grade and a serious student. Although she's a quiet girl, she enjoys an active social life and has a lot of friends. Sonia and her family are amazingly resilient; not only have they mastered a new language and become integrated into a new culture in the past year and a half, they are also well on their way to mastering Sonia's newly diagnosed diabetes.

For each of these youngsters and their families, diabetes, and all that goes with it, is a challenge that they are forced to meet each and every day. With each milestone in life, a new aspect of living with diabetes is revealed. Indeed, the immediate and long-term health and emotional well-being of the child, and to some extent of the entire family, depend on the successful integration of diabetes into their lives.

What exactly is diabetes? What is involved in "managing" or "controlling" diabetes? How do growth and development affect diabetes and, conversely, how does diabetes impact on growth and development? This book addresses these and many other questions, so that friends and relatives, health care professionals, teachers,

coaches, school bus drivers and camp counselors can more effectively support children and their families as they embark on a life's
journey with diabetes.

The information and insights presented here will interest both
those who are new to diabetes in young people, and those who
are experienced with it. Each phase of adapting to the disorder
and each stage of child and family development bring new questions, concerns and expectations related to diabetes management.
Families and care providers will find this book an excellent
resource, but it has its limitations. It cannot and should not replace
the comprehensive education program provided to the child and
family, at the time of diagnosis and beyond, by a team of experienced health professionals.

Gathering together the collected wisdom of the pediatric diabetes team, including children, adolescents and their families, this
is a practical guide for young people with diabetes, their families,
and everyone else who cares about them.

The Diabetes Team

To meet the complex and ever-changing demands of living with
diabetes, all children, teens and their families should have access
to and be able to work with an experienced diabetes health care
team. Each professional in this group brings unique experience
and expertise to the care of the child or teen and the support
of the family. At the center of this interdisciplinary team,
however, are the child and the family, because care must be tai-
lored to meet their individual needs. The "core" team should
also include:

- a physician, usually a pediatric endocrinologist or diabetologist
- a diabetes nurse (often called a diabetes nurse educator)
- a diabetes dietitian
- a social worker or counselor

Members of the "extended" team, in addition to other family members, include:
- the family practitioner or pediatrician
- school personnel
- recreation workers
- the pharmacist
- babysitters
- others who share responsibility for child care and/or supporting the family

The diabetes team

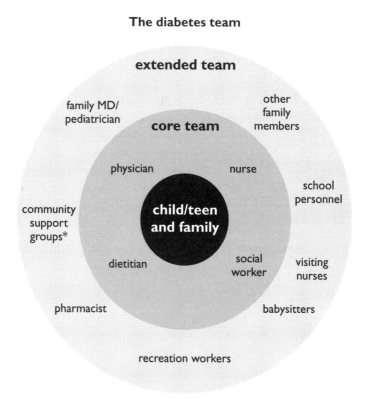

* such as American Diabetes Association,
Canadian Diabetes Association,
Juvenile Diabetes Foundation

What Do You Need to Learn and Why?

In the following chapters we will answer these important questions:

- What happens when someone develops diabetes?
- What does "blood glucose balance" mean and what affects it?
- What do we need to know about insulin?
- Why do we need a meal plan?
- How do we assess the effectiveness of diabetes care routines?
- What do we do when blood glucose is out of balance?
- How do we deal with the emotional impact of diabetes?
- How does diabetes care differ at different ages?
- Do we need to worry about diabetes complications?
- Will the child become a healthy adult?
- What is the future of diabetes?

Diabetes at any age is a real challenge. It imposes itself on virtually all aspects of daily life. Learning about diabetes, and how to manage or control it, is essential so that children and teens can get on with their lives with as little risk and as much vigor as possible. Read on and learn.

O N E

Overview

It had been a hot and humid summer. Jim and Ruth didn't think it was terribly unusual that their eight-year-old son, Danny, seemed to be drinking so much water. They also felt that, since he was drinking so much, it was normal for him to get up a couple of times each night to urinate. What started to worry them was the weight loss: in June he had weighed 56 pounds (25 kg) at his annual checkup, and now, in mid-July, he looked skinny and weighed in at only 49 pounds (22 kg). The neighbors said not to worry—it was summer, and Danny was burning up so much energy at day camp that the weight loss was just part of his normal development.

Ruth's concern reached a crisis point when Danny started to feel listless and vomited three times one Sunday morning. Jim was out of town on business, so it was Ruth's decision to head to the hospital to see what was going on.

The doctors and nurses in the emergency room seemed to pick up the clues right away: the increased urination and thirst, coupled with weight loss, and now vomiting and dehydration, all pointed to diabetes. They confirmed their suspicions with a quick urine check and blood tests; both showed high amounts of sugar. Danny was admitted and immediately given an intravenous drip to replace fluids, and the hormone insulin, which would help deal with the excess sugar. Within hours, he began to look more like his former self and was feeling much better. By the next morning he was well enough to be taken off the intravenous and receive his first insulin injection before breakfast. His father returned quickly from his business trip. It was time for the family to begin to learn the ropes of living with diabetes.

What Is Diabetes?

To a child with diabetes, the very first syllable of the word can seem frightening. Younger children think in very concrete terms, and many wonder if a person with "die"abetes is going to die. But the word "diabetes" comes from the Greek word for "to run through" or "to siphon." Diabetes has been known since about 1500 B.C., when the first medical document referring to excessive urine production was written. Sometime between 30 B.C. and A.D. 45, Aretacus of Cappadocia, a Greek physician, applied the term to people who had to urinate frequently. When doctors in the seventeenth century further discovered that the urine was sweet, they added the Latin word *mellitus*, meaning honey. In fact, an early method of diagnosis was to pour the urine on the ground; if ants scurried to the site, the doctor's suspicion was confirmed.

People lose sugar in their urine when they are missing the essential hormone *insulin*. A hormone is a chemical "messenger" that travels from one part of the body to tell another part what to do. Only with the help of insulin can the body's metabolic processes release the energy from the sugar in the food we eat, to let our muscles work, to produce our body heat, and for the continual growth, renewal and repair of the billions of cells that make up our bodies. (Metabolic processes are the complex series of chemical reactions that work to either produce or employ energy for the functioning of the body.) Without insulin, we can't survive.

The digestive system

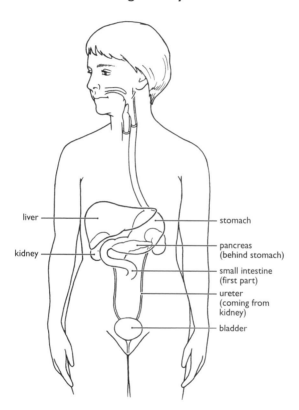

liver — stomach

kidney — pancreas (behind stomach)

small intestine (first part)

ureter (coming from kidney)

bladder

Insulin is made in the pancreas (an organ located just behind the stomach) by highly specialized cells known as *beta cells*. These are found within the pancreas, in islands of tissue named the islets of Langerhans, for the scientist, Paul Langerhans, who discovered them.

In children and teens with diabetes, the beta cells have been destroyed. This means that insulin can no longer be produced. The only way they can once again use sugar for energy is to replace the missing insulin, and at present this can only be done effectively by daily insulin injections. When children develop diabetes, only the insulin-producing cells are destroyed. The rest of the pancreas is healthy and continues to produce digestive enzymes and another hormone called *glucagon*.

The pancreas

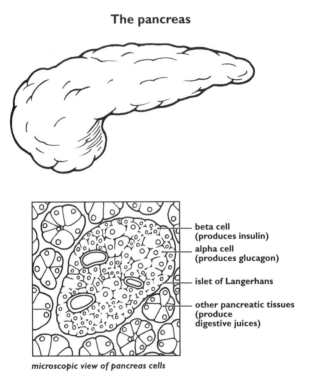

microscopic view of pancreas cells

This inability to produce any insulin is characteristic of Type 1 diabetes. Most people with diabetes are adults and have Type 2 diabetes, which means that they can produce some insulin but it doesn't work properly to use up all the available sugar.

Types of Diabetes

Most people know somebody with diabetes. Friends and colleagues are quick to offer well-meaning advice about their 50-year-old uncle who was recently diagnosed with diabetes, or their sister who had diabetes while she was pregnant. They tell stories of people who had to cut out sweets and trim fat from their diets, take medication and exercise, but didn't require daily insulin injections. Then why do children with diabetes require insulin injections?

Simply, because of the different kinds of diabetes. Children almost always have Type 1—previously known as insulin-dependent diabetes mellitus (IDDM), or juvenile diabetes. In Type 1 diabetes, the pancreas loses its ability to produce any or enough insulin. By the time the symptoms of the disorder have developed, at least 80 percent of the beta cells have already been destroyed. Nobody knows for certain how long this destruction has been progressing but it is probably many months or years. Type 1 diabetes is usually diagnosed before age forty, and most commonly in children aged two to sixteen. Of all the people with diabetes in North America, Type 1 affects only 10 percent. Of that 10 percent, half are under the age of twenty.

The rest of the diabetes population has Type 2 diabetes, or non-insulin-dependent diabetes mellitus (NIDDM). The beta cells are still present in the pancreas, but either they don't make enough insulin, or the insulin they produce doesn't work well enough to keep blood sugar levels normal. This occurs most often in overweight adults. The first line of treatment is strict dietary management and attention to lifestyle issues such as doing more exercise and quitting smoking. In addition to diet, an oral medication may be used to help the pancreas make more insulin or to make the insulin work better. Sometimes the doctor

Types of diabetes

	Type 1	Type 2
also called	insulin-dependent diabetes mellitus (IDDM) juvenile diabetes childhood diabetes	non-insulin-dependent diabetes mellitus (NIDDM) maturity-onset diabetes adult-onset diabetes
usually diagnosed in	younger people (between infancy and 40)	older people (over 40; incidence increases with age); often people with a significant weight problem
insulin is	eventually totally absent	produced, but too little or too ineffective to deal with the demands of the body
accounts for	about 10% of all people with diabetes	90% of all people with diabetes
is treated by	insulin injections (plus a meal plan and careful monitoring)	diet first to reduce weight; oral medications to either stimulate more insulin production or make the available insulin work better; or insulin, if the first two methods are unsuccessful

will also prescribe insulin injections for people with Type 2 diabetes, but this doesn't change the diagnosis to Type 1.

Some women develop diabetes during pregnancy. This is known as *gestational diabetes*. Women with gestational diabetes need the help of an expert team to achieve excellent blood sugar control, to give them the best possible chance of having a healthy baby. Treatment involves careful monitoring, some changes in meal planning and in some cases insulin injections. After the baby is born, the mother's pancreas usually begins functioning normally again. Although the infants of mothers with gestational diabetes are no more likely to develop diabetes than any other babies, women who have had gestational diabetes are at increased risk of developing Type 2 diabetes later in life.

What Causes Type 1 Diabetes?

We do not know exactly why otherwise healthy people develop diabetes, but research has given us some clues. Type 1 diabetes is an autoimmune disorder, much like many thyroid disorders, rheumatoid arthritis, lupus or multiple sclerosis. In these diseases, the body starts to see a part of itself as "foreign" and the immune system responds by destroying certain cells. In diabetes, the immune system destroys the insulin-producing beta cells. Researchers have so far identified two main factors behind this autoimmune response:

Genetics

It appears that the susceptibility to develop Type 1 diabetes is inherited, rather than the disease itself. This means that only some people born with a high level of susceptibility will actually develop the disorder. In fact, we find a history of other family members with Type 1 diabetes in less than 10 percent of families. The fact that genetic factors can't be used to predict diabetes with 100 percent certainty suggests that other, presumably environmental factors may also be involved.

Environment

The exact environmental trigger or triggers responsible for diabetes have not yet been determined. Some researchers believe that certain viral infections, illnesses or environmental

Risk of developing Type 1 diabetes if a family member has it

Sibling (including non-identical twin)	1 in 20 chance
Identical twin	1 in 2–3 chance
Mother	1 in 50–100 chance
Father	1 in 16–20 chance
No family member	1 in 250–400 chance

or food toxins may either damage the pancreas directly or trigger the autoimmune response. Many children diagnosed with diabetes have recently recovered from a virus or other illness. But everyone gets viruses and very few get diabetes. Although high levels of stress or even the onset of puberty frequently precedes the development of diabetes, stress is not generally believed to be the cause.

While diabetes is an autoimmune disorder, children with diabetes are no more susceptible to illness than any other child. Some people who have no personal experience of diabetes may be afraid that it's contagious, or may think of a child with diabetes as being "sick." Diabetes is not contagious. It cannot be passed on to another person through sharing a drink, playing together, kissing or in any other way. Children with diabetes are just as healthy as their friends without it, once they have begun to manage the disease.

It's human nature to want to assign blame when something goes wrong. Many parents—and even children—are quick to blame the diabetes on themselves. Women sometimes fear they didn't take good enough care of themselves while pregnant; some worry their child ate too many sweets. But research shows that parents can't do anything to either cause or prevent diabetes. Nor can children. Children aren't born with Type 1 diabetes, and at this stage we cannot yet predict with certainty who is going to get the disorder. And even if we could predict it, we would still have no way to prevent its onset.

What Does Insulin Do?
How does insulin work with food? In a nutshell, here's what happens.

When we eat, the food goes to the stomach and the small intestines, where it is digested or broken down into components, or nutrients, small enough to be absorbed into the bloodstream and carried to every part of the body.

Food consists of three main nutrients: carbohydrate, protein and fat. Our bodies derive energy from all three. Through digestion, carbohydrates (such as those in bread, potatoes and fruit) are broken down into sugar, or *glucose*; proteins (in foods such as meat and cheese) are converted into *amino acids*; and fats, including butter and oils, turn into *fatty acids*.

Glucose is an especially important source of energy, for two reasons: it can be converted quickly into energy when we need it, such as during work or sports; and the brain and nerves rely on a constant supply of glucose for their function.

In response to the glucose entering the bloodstream, the pancreas secretes insulin into the blood. Insulin stimulates the uptake of glucose by all the cells of the body, so that they have the energy to do their work. Insulin also allows excess sugar to be stored in the liver, in the form of *glycogen*, or deposited in fat cells, where it becomes another important source of stored energy.

The insulin secreted by the pancreas in response to a meal is just the right amount to keep the blood sugar from going too high. After most of the nutrients from the meal have been taken up by the cells and the blood glucose concentration once again approaches "fasting" levels, the pancreas secretes less insulin into the blood.

A little bit of insulin (called a *basal amount*) is almost always being produced by our bodies. This is needed because, between meals and while we sleep, the liver continues to release some of its stored sugar into the blood, so that our brain and nerves receive the constant supply of glucose that they need to survive.

Turning food into energy: without diabetes

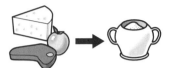

The stomach turns food into sugar.

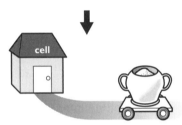

The sugar is carried through the blood.

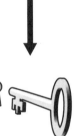

The pancreas makes enough
insulin to open the cell door.

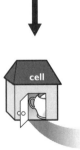

Sugar enters the cell,
where it is used to make energy.

Turning food into energy: with diabetes

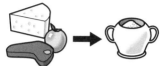

The stomach turns food into sugar.

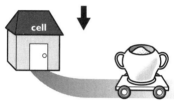

The sugar is carried through the blood.

without insulin	with insulin

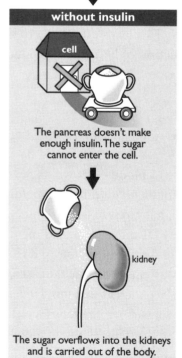

The pancreas doesn't make enough insulin. The sugar cannot enter the cell.

kidney

The sugar overflows into the kidneys and is carried out of the body.

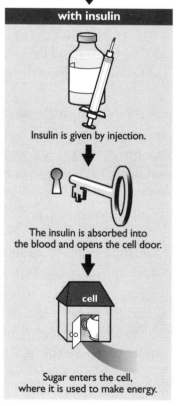

Insulin is given by injection.

The insulin is absorbed into the blood and opens the cell door.

Sugar enters the cell, where it is used to make energy.

This basal amount of insulin ensures that the balance between the amount of glucose being produced by the liver, and that being used by the cells of the body, is perfectly maintained to prevent either low or high glucose levels.

Later, when we eat again, another burst of insulin is secreted from the pancreas into the blood, and the liver stops releasing stored sugar and begins to replenish its stores for later use.

In summary: Insulin is an essential hormone. It acts as a key opening the door to the body cells, allowing glucose to enter and to be used to make the energy so vital to their function. Without enough insulin, sugar cannot be taken up and used by most of the body cells. The cells starve, even though the blood glucose concentration may be very high, and the body seeks alternate sources of energy. This leads eventually to the breakdown of fat and the production of harmful byproducts called *ketones* (see below).

Normal Blood Sugar Regulation

If someone without diabetes were to measure blood sugar before breakfast (called *fasting blood sugar*), it would be 3.3 to 6 millimoles of sugar per liter of blood—known as 3.3 to 6 mmol/L (about 60–110 milligrams per deciliter or mg/dL). After eating, sugar levels will rise, but rarely above 8.9 mmol/L or 160 mg/dL, and never above 11.1 mmol/L or 200 mg/dL. Very small amounts of insulin are continuously released from the healthy pancreas. As soon as the blood sugar rises, a message goes to the beta cells in the pancreas that more insulin is required. The beta cells have sensors on their surface that detect the blood sugar level and give out just the right amount of insulin to handle the increased blood sugar.

When the blood sugar level comes down again, the burst of extra insulin shuts off. The beta cells keep a reserve of insulin on hand, and when that is used up, they produce more. So the next time the person eats—be it a four-course meal or a quick snack—the pancreas responds with just the right amount of insulin to bring the blood sugar level back into fasting range. This system works so efficiently in people without diabetes that, regardless of how much they eat, or how long they go without food, the blood sugar remains within the normal range. If a person doesn't eat at all, the extra insulin just doesn't turn on. Other hormones—such as glucagon, which is also made in the pancreas—kick in to keep the blood sugar from going too low.

What Happens in Children Who Aren't Making or Taking Any Insulin?

As the child with diabetes eats, the food still releases sugar in the process of digestion. This sugar is absorbed into the bloodstream and is carried to the cells. But the pancreas doesn't respond by making insulin, so the sugar can't move *into* the cells. When the sugar remains locked out of the cells, a chain of events is set in motion. The child may become tired, because the cells are literally starved for energy. Meanwhile, sugar continues to build up in the blood. If this were allowed to continue, the blood would eventually become so thick and syrupy that it wouldn't flow through the veins. Fortunately, the kidneys do their job—to filter blood and eliminate, through the urine, substances that might otherwise harm the body.

When the kidneys sense a high level of sugar in the blood, they start eliminating it via the urine. The point at which the kidneys allow sugar to enter the urine is called the *renal* (kidney) *threshold*. When this excess sugar is eliminated, it takes with it the water in which it is dissolved, so the child urinates more often and in larger amounts (*polyuria*) just to get rid of the sugar. The higher the blood sugar level, the more frequent the urination. Increased urination leads to dehydration, so the body demands more water, and the child becomes increasingly thirsty (*polydipsia*). Children may complain of a dry sticky mouth or sore dry throat. Parents report children gulping down jugs of juice, and quarts of milk or water. Sometimes parents think the increased urination is caused by the excessive drinking, so they try to cut off the fluids. However, the child continues to urinate frequently, because the body's priority is to clear out the sugar. Drinking all this fluid is the only way the child can avoid dehydration.

Excessive urination and thirst are usually the first indications of the high blood sugar (*hyperglycemia*) of diabetes. Some children have to get up in the middle of the night to go to the bathroom (*nocturia*). Younger children may even start wetting the bed (*enuresis*). The loss of sugar in the urine, together with dehydration and the inability to use blood sugar, can lead to weight loss despite an increase in appetite (*polyphagia*). As the symptoms develop, children often feel tired, drowsy and weak.

Using Fat for Energy
When Danny was admitted to hospital, his body was unable to make any, or enough, insulin to use sugar as energy. So where was he getting his energy? When the pancreas doesn't make insulin and the cells don't get their energy, the body starts to break down fat and proteins to be used as energy. When the body breaks down fat, there is weight loss, which accounted for Danny's gaunt appearance. In the process of breaking down fat for energy, the body makes a potentially poisonous byproduct called ketones, or acetone—the same chemical used in nailpolish remover.

As soon as ketones are made, the kidneys recognize that they are poisonous and filter them out through the urine. Because Ruth didn't know her son had diabetes, she had no way of knowing that there were ketones present, or even what ketones were. Soon, Danny couldn't filter out the ketones as fast as they were being made, and they began to build up in his blood, leading to his stomachaches and severe nausea. This buildup of ketones is called *diabetic ketoacidosis (DKA)*. When the body can't get rid of all the ketones through the urine, it can even resort to exhaling them, so that a fruity or unnatural smell may be noticeable on the child's breath. Danny's heavy, rapid breathing was his body's attempt to get rid of more ketones. This is called *Kussmaul breathing*.

Ketoacidosis is a serious condition that can lead to unconsciousness and death. Fortunately, giving intravenous fluid and insulin corrects the situation. In fact, this is the sickest most children with diabetes will ever be. Once a child has been diagnosed with diabetes, and the parents gain the tools and support they need to manage the disorder, diabetic ketoacidosis should be totally avoidable. Today diabetes is most often diagnosed before DKA has developed. The presence of the classic symptoms of diabetes should trigger further investigation.

While these symptoms may be clear in older children, they may be less obvious in infants and toddlers. It's difficult to

---

Early symptoms of untreated or undiagnosed diabetes

Children with diabetes may:
* urinate a lot and often
* feel thirsty
* feel tired
* lose weight despite increased appetite

recognize thirst in young children who cannot speak. And regular growth spurts can bring changes in appetite. In these cases, therefore, the condition may quickly progress to DKA before it is recognized. An additional sign in those still in diapers may be a fungal or yeast diaper rash that doesn't improve with the use of medicated cream. These organisms flourish in the sugar excreted in the urine. In older girls, yeast infections (for example, vaginal discharge or itching) may also precede diagnosis.

Confirming the Diagnosis

Danny's parents could hardly believe that, with one urine test and one blood test, their son was sentenced to a life of injections. They thought that surely such a devastating diagnosis required a battery of tests to rule out other possibilities. The simple truth is that a urine test showing a lot of sugar as well as the presence of ketones, accompanied by symptoms such as excessive thirst and urination, establishes the diagnosis of diabetes. A reliable laboratory blood sugar reading of more than 11.1 mmol/L (200 mg/dL) taken at any time of day, regardless of when the child last ate, confirms it.

In children, making the distinction between Type 1 and Type 2 diabetes is usually not difficult. By far the majority of children and teens have Type 1. Symptoms of Type 1 diabetes usually have a dramatic onset because the pancreas stops making insulin at all. Ketones are much more likely to be present in the urine in Type 1 diabetes than in Type 2. However, the absence of ketones doesn't mean that it isn't Type 1; rather, it suggests that the child was diagnosed early, before ketones had the chance to form. Unfortunately, early diagnosis doesn't mean a milder course of treatment, or mean that the child will have a less severe case of diabetes.

The child's symptoms disappear quite quickly once the insulin is replaced by injection. A few weeks after diagnosis, many parents are surprised to find that the insulin requirement decreases, giving the impression that the diabetes is going away. This is known as the remission, or the *honeymoon period*. During this time, the pancreas seems to be able to secrete some insulin, but this is only temporary. These changes in insulin need do not mean that the diabetes was misdiagnosed or that it has been cured. This period can last a few months or even a year or longer, but during that time the pancreas continues to lose insulin-producing cells. As the honeymoon comes to an end, the blood sugar rises and the daily insulin dose should increase, usually gradually, to an amount more consistent with what a child of that particular height and weight would require. This increase in insulin requirement should be seen as part of the natural course of the disease, rather than an indication that the diabetes is suddenly "getting worse."

Type 2 Diabetes in Children and Adolescents

Although Type 2 diabetes is much less common in children and adolescents, there is some indication that it is increasing in frequency. Type 2 diabetes is much more likely to be found in adolescents than in younger children.

Certain risk factors predispose young people to the development of Type 2 diabetes. These include:

- a strong family history of Type 2 diabetes, especially if it developed in other family members at a young age;
- obesity;
- being a member of an ethnic group or population known to have a much higher prevalence of Type 2 diabetes, such as African American and African Canadian, aboriginal American and aboriginal Canadian, or Hispanic.

As explained earlier, Type 2 diabetes results from a combination of impaired insulin action in the muscle and fat cells of the body, and decreased insulin secretion from the pancreas. It is often associated with high blood fat (cholesterol and triglycerides) levels, high blood pressure and a serious risk of later cardiovascular disease (heart attack or stroke).

Although the majority of adolescents with Type 2 diabetes are considerably overweight, there are some who are thin, and the latter often have a strong family history of thin relatives developing Type 2 diabetes at a young age. This type of diabetes is inherited as a dominant condition (that is, parents who have it may pass it on directly to half their children), and is called Maturity Onset Diabetes in the Young, or MODY.

In comparison to Type 1 diabetes, Type 2 diabetes usually begins with much milder symptoms, or without any symptoms at all. Occasionally, there is diabetic ketoacidosis (DKA), which can confuse the diagnosis.

The diagnosis of Type 2 diabetes in adolescents is usually made after Type 1 has been ruled out. If the young person has a strong history of symptoms, very high blood sugar readings and ketones in the urine, Type 1 diabetes is diagnosed. In an older adolescent with elevated blood glucose and only mild (or no) symptoms and no urinary ketones, Type 2 diabetes is a possibility, but so is the early phase of Type 1. Sometimes the doctor requests a blood test for islet cell antibodies. A positive result indicates Type 1 diabetes; a negative result is inconclusive.

The initial management of Type 2 diabetes depends on the blood sugar level and the severity of symptoms. Careful attention to meal planning is the cornerstone of treatment, and sometimes diet is enough to control the blood sugar. Of course, for an obese teen with Type 2 diabetes an important goal of nutritional management is weight loss, which can be difficult. These young people need the help of a dietitian who understands adolescents, as well as a supportive family environment. If diet alone does not adequately control the blood glucose levels over the long term, medication may be required. Unlike Type 1 diabetes, in which pills are of no benefit, in Type 2, oral hypoglycemic agents (pills) such as sulphonylureas or biguanides are sometimes effective. These agents either stimulate the pancreas to produce more insulin, or help the cells of the body respond better to the insulin available. If blood sugar cannot be controlled with these agents, insulin treatment is necessary.

For young people who have more severe symptoms and higher blood sugar readings, it is usually necessary to start with insulin and then reconsider, as the diabetes progresses, whether oral hypoglycemic agents may be helpful.

This book focuses on the care of children and adolescents with Type 1 diabetes. Although many of the concepts discussed apply to both types, young people diagnosed with Type 2 diabetes should discuss possible differences, such as the role of exercise and the timing of meals, with their health care team.

Q&A

If the pancreas isn't working anymore, should it be removed?
No. Even if the beta cells are not producing insulin, the rest of the pancreas is still healthy and working. It is not a diseased organ, nor will it hinder the body in any other way. We know this because the pancreas also releases enzyme-rich juices that aid in digestion, and children or teens with diabetes do not experience any unusual digestive problems. It also produces other hormones, such as glucagon, which may help protect against hypoglycemia.

Why can't insulin be administered by mouth?
Insulin is a protein hormone. Taken as a tablet or liquid, it would be broken down and digested in the stomach. However, insulin can't act unless it reaches the bloodstream before it's broken down. Therefore, it must be injected with a needle and syringe under the skin into an area of body fat. From there it is gradually absorbed into the bloodstream and transported to the cells.

When my uncle had a heart attack, the doctors discovered he had diabetes. He was on insulin for four or five years. Then, once he got his blood sugar under control, he didn't have to take it anymore. Is there a possibility my child might not need to take insulin after a while?
Unfortunately, there is no known cure for Type 1 diabetes, and insulin injections remain the only way to manage it. Some people with Type 2 diabetes, like your uncle, go on insulin to gain tighter control of their blood sugar during a particularly stressful period (such as after a heart attack) or until they've lost some weight. Eventually they may be able to keep good blood sugar control with diet alone or with pills.

My child has had diabetes for three weeks now, and it seems that our whole lives revolve around the disease. Is this going to go on forever?
The way you're feeling right now is normal and necessary. Learning about diabetes, and adjusting to it, should be your priority. The immediate impact of the disorder is overwhelming for all members of the family. Try to take one day at a time, and don't be afraid to lean on your diabetes team for support and guidance. As time goes on, you will feel more comfortable with the daily routines of diabetes care. But be

patient; it can take a year or perhaps longer before you go a day without worrying about your child's condition.

How will I know if one of my other children is developing diabetes?
The table earlier in the chapter shows the likelihood of others in the family developing diabetes. If this should happen in one of your other children, he or she will almost certainly start to show such "classic" symptoms as increased urination and thirst, and weight loss. If you are concerned, simply do a urine test for sugar. If there is no sugar present, it's not diabetes. If there is sugar present, contact your family doctor or diabetes team.

What do I say when people ask why I was away from school?
It's often difficult for children to know what and when to tell classmates. Other children may be scared, too. Tell them that diabetes is *not* contagious. To anyone who wants to know more, or anyone with whom you wish to share your condition, you can say that diabetes simply means that your body needs help making energy from your food. You need to take insulin injections because your body stopped making its own insulin. Involve your friends in your diabetes routines, if they want to learn and if you are comfortable showing them. You may even want to prepare a presentation or science project about diabetes.

Striking a Balance

Phil and Arlene are very proud of their daughter Jenny. At age 14, just one year after being diagnosed with diabetes, Jenny has taken on many of the responsibilities of monitoring and treating her own condition. She checks her blood sugar four times a day, prepares and injects her needles, and follows her daily meal plan by eating similar amounts of food at about the same times every day. Every night Arlene checks Jenny's diabetes log to make sure she's keeping track. Jenny carefully records how much insulin she takes and when, and color-codes the results of her glucose tests according to the level: red for over 8 mmol/L (145 mg/dL); green for her target range of 4 to 8 mmol/L; and blue for under 4 mmol/L (70 mg/dL). The logbook pages of the past month are mostly green, except for a few numbers in red and three or four in blue.

Jenny has had no low blood sugar readings that she hasn't been able to handle. A couple of times she got shaky after a rigorous game of soccer. Fortunately, she remembered to boost her blood sugar with a little juice (she always carries a juice box in her knapsack) and she felt fine after just a couple of minutes.

Jenny loves school too much to miss it, and her teacher recently commented that she hadn't thought about Jenny's diabetes in months. Arlene wishes she could say the same. Even though she worries less about Jenny now than during those first few months, it's always in the back of her mind. Jenny has diabetes. Arlene has to remind herself that, unless medical science finds a way to overcome the disease, Jenny will always have diabetes.

Balanced blood sugar

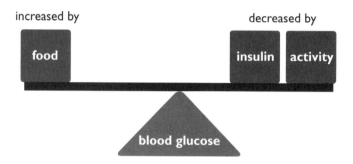

The Concept of Blood Glucose Balance

Blood glucose levels go up and down throughout the day. Think of a teeter-totter. When you eat, blood glucose goes up. When you exercise, blood glucose goes down. In people without diabetes, insulin automatically accommodates these fluctuations. People with diabetes inject insulin in an attempt to mimic the body's natural insulin action as closely as possible. However, injected insulin cannot perfectly match the fluctuations in blood sugar, so someone with diabetes has to work constantly to keep the teeter-totter from tipping.

The goal of diabetes management is to restore and maintain balance. The first step is to eliminate any symptoms of high blood sugar with insulin injections. The next step is to match the child's appetite and dietary needs for growth and development with the amount of insulin injected. As children grow and develop and their lifestyle and activities change, so do their insulin needs.

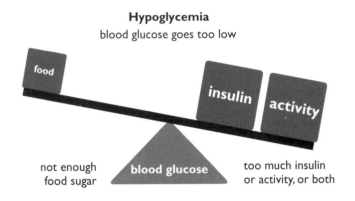

Hypoglycemia
blood glucose goes too low

not enough
food sugar

too much insulin
or activity, or both

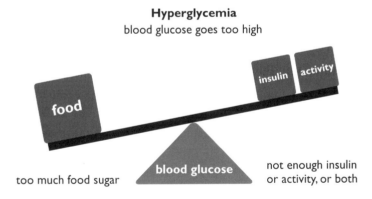

Hyperglycemia
blood glucose goes too high

too much food sugar

not enough insulin
or activity, or both

Blood glucose balance is important to immediate and long-term health. There are two immediate consequences of blood sugar imbalance. If the blood sugar level dips too low (usually below 3–4 mmol/L or 55–70 mg/dL), the child can become shaky, hungry, tired or grouchy. Eventually, if no sugar is given, the child may become confused or unconscious. This is called hypoglycemia. If the blood sugar level climbs too high (usually above 11 mmol/L, or 200 mg/dL), symptoms such as frequent urination and excessive thirst may recur. This is called hyperglycemia. Left untreated, hyperglycemia and insulin deficiency can lead to ketone production and eventually diabetic ketoacidosis.

Paying close attention to the blood sugar balance day after day is hard work. But over the long run, it's worth it. In 1993 the results of a landmark nine-year study, the Diabetes Control and Complications Trial (DCCT), showed that good blood sugar control over time makes a difference to future health. The better the control, the less likely the development of long-term complications to eyes, kidneys and nerves. We'll talk more about these risks in Chapter Nine.

Most young children and adolescents are unmoved by the threat of long-term complications, and indeed these complications are unheard of in children and extremely rare even in teens. But establishing good health care habits from the beginning will go a long way toward decreasing the risk of complications in adulthood.

Education is the cornerstone of managing diabetes. Learning as much as you can about diabetes and how to manage it will help you feel more secure, and will alleviate your fears and concerns. The goal of diabetes management is to help children live long, healthy, productive lives, as much like any other child as possible.

Gaining Control

Before looking down the road into adulthood, children with diabetes and their parents need to figure out how to live with diabetes from day to day. People with "good diabetes control" should expect to have general physical and emotional well-being, characterized by:

- no symptoms of high blood sugar levels (i.e. increased urination and thirst)
- only mild and infrequent low blood sugar reactions
- normal growth and physical development
- lots of energy
- interest in friends and activities
- regular school attendance

Factors That Affect Blood Glucose Balance

Insulin and food have a major impact on blood sugar level. The carbohydrates in the food we eat increase our blood sugar. Insulin lowers the blood sugar level by allowing sugar to enter the cells, where it's used for energy. For people with Type 1 diabetes, daily insulin injections and meal plans are the most important tools for keeping blood glucose in balance.

Insulin

In people without diabetes, the pancreas delivers insulin continuously throughout the day, then secretes extra insulin when food enters the system in order to counteract the increase in blood glucose. Injected insulin performs a similar function. Young children may start out with two or three injections of insulin each day (before breakfast, supper and bed). Older children and adolescents may take three or four. More frequent injections make sense in many ways, since this pattern more closely imitates the natural insulin supply.

Food

To achieve blood sugar balance, it's important for children to eat similar amounts of food at the same time each day. This is necessary because the insulin is intended to balance the glucose from food; it's impossible to know how much insulin to take if the timing and size of meals and snacks vary from day to day. If there isn't enough glucose in the body to work with the insulin, the child runs the risk of hypoglycemia and a subsequent insulin reaction. Conversely, if there is too much food for the given amount of insulin, hyperglycemia will result.

Most parents agree that this is the biggest challenge in managing diabetes. A dietitian will help devise a meal plan, keeping family habits and favorite foods in mind. The goal is *not* to restrict food or calories, but to ensure healthy eating and to help determine the insulin dosage.

Other Factors Affecting Glucose Control

We talk about insulin and meal plans so much because the child and parents have control over how much insulin is taken and how much food is eaten. But no matter how hard you try to match a consistent diet with the prescribed insulin regimen, the results of the blood sugar readings will vary. Why? Injected insulin can't match the automatic response of a normal pancreas. And there are other factors that affect blood glucose which are difficult to control, particularly in children, such as activity and stress.

Activity

Activity in the presence of insulin lowers the blood sugar level, because when the body burns more energy it uses more sugar. An active lifestyle is an important aspect of good health. It improves physical fitness, helps us relax and promotes general well-being. A child's diabetes care routine should take into account the amount of exercise or activity he or she experiences on a daily basis. Parents, and eventually the child, will learn to adjust the routines for special activities.

For people with diabetes, exercise offers an additional

advantage. It helps improve the action of a given amount of insulin, so that less insulin may be needed to maintain the blood sugar level. For example, an active person requires less insulin than someone watching television, because activity brings blood glucose down. Regular exercise also seems to make muscles and other tissues more receptive to insulin, so the body requires less insulin to move glucose from the blood into the muscles. As well, regular exercise may help decrease the risk of diabetes complications.

These benefits aside, exercise and activity must not be considered a tool of diabetes treatment. Children generally lead naturally active lives; turning exercise into something "prescribed" takes the fun away. A positive example from parents is essential. Exercise and activity should be part of an enjoyable family routine. That's not to say that everyone with diabetes has to become a competitive athlete, but children should participate in sports and physical activity at their own level.

How Exercise Affects Blood Sugar

In general, activity causes the muscles to draw more glucose from the blood. In people without diabetes, the pancreas makes and secretes much less insulin, the liver produces more glucose for the body to use and the level of glucose in the blood remains steady.

In children with diabetes, the injected insulin is unable to "shut off." The muscles continue to use up the available glucose in the blood. If the insulin is injected into an arm or leg in someone who has been particularly active, such as playing tag or bicycling, there may in fact be an increase in the flow of insulin absorbed from the injection site into the blood. This insulin causes the muscles to draw more glucose, prevents the liver from replenishing the supply of glucose in the blood, and may therefore put the child at risk of a low blood sugar reaction.

While most activities lead to a decrease in blood glucose levels, some very stressful or competitive activities (such as ice hockey or soccer) may increase the glucose levels, because the heavy stress of the game increases "stress" hormones that work against the insulin. Sometimes, too, the glucose level doesn't fall during the activity, especially if it occurs immediately after a meal. However, the glucose may then drop for up to six to twelve hours after the activity is over. This means that children doing strenuous activity in the late evening are susceptible to late-night "lows."

The diabetes team will help the family tailor their routine to the child's everyday activity. Precautions should be taken for extra, out-of-the-ordinary activities.

Stress

Stress generally increases the blood sugar level. Stress is the body's physical response to danger, left over from the days when we had to fight natural predators for survival. Though the causes of stress may have changed over the ages, the body's reaction hasn't. Stress triggers a surge of power-boosting hormones, such as adrenaline and glucagon. These hormones in turn stimulate a release of stored sugar into the blood. Children with diabetes do not automatically make more insulin to deal with this.

Today's stress can be emotional, caused by exams or peer pressure, for example, or physical, accompanying fever and infection. Stress can also come in the form of excitement over seeing friends and family, or anticipating a special occasion. The bottom line is that sometimes stress makes the blood sugar go up temporarily. During a stressful event like an illness, parents and child will need to check blood sugar levels more frequently and take appropriate action.

Parents do not need to make any special attempt to create a "stress-free" environment for their child. Checking blood sugar regularly and making adjustments based on the results will help maintain the blood sugar balance.

Checking Blood Glucose Balance

Checking blood glucose levels several times each day is the best way to determine how well the child with diabetes is balancing insulin, food and activity.

The diabetes health care team works with the family to determine a blood sugar range that fits each child's age and stage of development. No matter how hard the parents and child try to monitor meals and snacks, or how carefully they stick to insulin regimens and activities, not every reading will fall into this range. In the beginning, very few may. It is not unusual for parents or children to feel they have done something "wrong" or "bad" if levels are off target. Avoid looking at each blood sugar check as a report card; rather, see it as a piece of a road map that helps you make appropriate decisions about diabetes management.

Q&A

I read somewhere that, after they're diagnosed with Type 1 diabetes, people can become overweight. Is this true?

Not really. When diabetes develops there is usually some weight loss (sometimes just a little, other times quite a lot). With treatment the lost weight will soon be regained. Otherwise, young people with Type 1 diabetes, particularly teenage girls, are only slightly more likely than their non-diabetic peers to become overweight.

My daughter isn't very active. I'd like to get her involved in something physical, to avoid increasing her insulin. What can you suggest?
It's great that you want to encourage your daughter to get more involved in physical fitness, but remember, exercise is not therapy. If she preferred books to baseball before she had diabetes, there's no reason to expect her to change now. As well, she may come to need more insulin to meet the demands of her growing body. All children require increased insulin until they finish growing. Nevertheless, encourage her to participate in physical activities. You might start with family walks and go on to other social activities she likes, such as bicycling, swimming or tennis.

Why doesn't exercise always help bring down high blood sugar?
In general, exercise does help lower the blood sugar level. But once blood glucose is very high—for example, over 17.0 mmol/L (300 mg/dL)—don't count on exercise to bring it down. The only thing sure to bring it down is insulin. Strenuous exercise without enough insulin prompts the liver to release stored sugar, which in turn increases blood glucose. In someone with high blood sugar and not enough insulin, the glucose just keeps building up. Don't exercise if you are ill and urine ketones are present.

Why does my son's blood sugar always go sky-high after exercise?
There are two reasons this may happen. First, if his diabetes is poorly controlled, so that he has frequent high blood sugar readings, exercise will be a further stress causing even higher sugar. Secondly, in some children with well-controlled diabetes, very strenuous exercise can cause stress and increased

glucose levels. They may not need extra food to cover the exercise, but may need more insulin. In such situations, beware of late-night lows.

My daughter was very sick with diabetic ketoacidosis at the time she was diagnosed. How can I be sure that she will never get sick like that again?
Once children are diagnosed with diabetes and established on insulin, there are really only two reasons why they might develop diabetic ketoacidosis again, and both are preventable. First, an illness such as a fever, infection or flu may create a demand for more insulin than normal. If you don't realize this and make the appropriate adjustments, DKA may result. We deal with illness management in Chapter Six.

Secondly, failure to take any or enough insulin will result in DKA. As long as you are in charge of giving the insulin, this is unlikely. However, when children are left to inject their own insulin unsupervised before they have developed sound judgment (or when an illness impairs their judgment), DKA may result when they forget, or even intentionally neglect, to inject the insulin. Wise parents remain involved in supporting and supervising their children with injections long into their adolescent years. As children become more independent, parents should watch for warning signs that things are not going well— for example, a recurrence of the symptoms of hyperglycemia or of ketones in the urine. When parents notice these signs they should resume close supervision, or even give the insulin injections for a while, regardless of their child's age.

THREE

All about Insulin

It has been six months since Margie was diagnosed with diabetes. She's a fun-loving, active four-year-old who has adjusted well, except to the insulin injections. She's great with the finger prick for blood sugar. She even applies the drop of blood to the strip. But when it comes to the injection, she kicks up a fuss. The shot before breakfast is especially hard for Margie and her parents, John and Liz. It's a hectic time: her brothers and sisters are busy getting ready for school, and Mom and Dad are trying to get off to work, and Margie throws a temper tantrum. John is just as happy to back off, since he hates giving Margie her injections anyway, which means Liz has to step in and get the needle over with. These episodes are wearing the family's patience thin, and not helping Margie either. "Try making it less of an ordeal," suggests their diabetes nurse when Liz calls in desperation one morning. "Draw the insulin, prepare the syringe and get everything ready before Margie even comes downstairs for breakfast." The nurse recommends that both John and Liz be present for the injection, to show Margie they are "there" for her, and to take some of the stress off Liz. It helps for one parent to hold Margie while the other gives the injection. Letting Margie hold a special stuffed toy may also comfort her.

Despite the long history of diabetes, no real headway was made in the understanding or treatment of the disease until 1889. German physiologists Oskar Minkowski and Joseph von Mering learned, quite accidentally, that the pancreas was central to diabetes. In studying digestion in a laboratory dog, they removed the pancreas to see the effect. When the dog started urinating more often than usual, the doctors tested the urine for sugar. Indeed, the dog had the markers of diabetes. In 1893, scientist Paul Langerhans isolated cells in the pancreas (the islets of Langerhans) that produced a hormone, but doctors still didn't understand its function.

As doctors inched closer to finding a treatment, young people with diabetes still didn't fare well. Most died within a year of diagnosis. In 1921 the breakthrough came, when a young surgeon at the University of Toronto, Dr. Frederick Banting, and his student, Charles Best, focused on the unknown hormone produced in the islets of Langerhans.

Still working with dogs, Banting and Best limited pancreatic function by tying off the ducts that send digestive enzymes from the pancreas into the intestine. The theory was that the islet cells, which secrete the hormone into the bloodstream, wouldn't be affected. Banting isolated a substance from these cells and injected it into a diabetic dog. The success was not immediate, but eventually Banting and Best treated the dog with the islet extract, soon to be labeled "insulin" (from the Latin word *insula*, meaning "island").

The real test, of course, was a human subject. Leonard Thompson, a 14-year-old boy dying of diabetes, was confined to his bed. He was little more than paper-thin skin wrapped around a skeleton. The first injection of insulin had no effect. A biochemist purified the canine insulin, and after 12 days of treatment the boy began to look like himself again. (Thompson eventually died of pneumonia at age 29.) Two years after their landmark discovery, Banting and Professor J.J.R. MacLeod (in whose lab the experiments took place) were awarded the Nobel Prize in Physiology and Medicine. Banting subsequently shared his prize with Best, while MacLeod recognized the efforts of the biochemist, J.B. Collip.

Types of Insulin
Initially manufacturers used cows and pigs to produce insulin. Pork insulin is still on the market, but since 1983 biosynthetic human insulin has been available. This is produced in a laboratory by introducing a synthetic human gene into bacteria or yeast, which produces insulin identical in structure and function to that created in the human pancreas. Through further modifications, manufacturers can prepare insulins with different action times. Although some people still use pork insulin, the majority now receive human insulin products.

Action
Manufactured insulin is generally categorized into three groups: fast-acting (also referred to as short-acting or rapid-acting), intermediate-acting and long-acting. Insulins are also described according to their course of action: *onset* is the time taken for the insulin to start working, *peak* describes the period when the insulin is working at its strongest and *duration* describes the length of time before the effect of the dose wears off. The newest development is superfast-acting insulin. Taken right before a meal, it begins to work within five to ten

Insulin's effect: how soon, how long

	Appearance	Onset	Peak	Duration
"Superfast" (Lispro)	clear	5–10 min.	first 2 hours	3–4 hours
Fast (Regular)	clear	1/2–1 hour	2–4 hours	4–6 hours
Intermediate (NPH or Lente)	cloudy	2–4 hours	6–12 hours	18–24 hours
Slow (Ultralente)	cloudy	4 hours	minimal peak	20–30 hours

(These times represent averages for each preparation, and may vary from person to person, from one injection site to another and to some extent in the same person from day to day. Lente insulin may have a slightly longer duration of action than NPH.)

minutes and helps to control the rise in blood sugar immediately after eating.

Insulin Strength

In North America insulin is dispensed in a concentration of 100 units/1 mL. It's available in bottles to be used with syringes, and in cartridges used with insulin pen injectors. Each bottle of insulin holds 10 mL, or 1,000 units. There are two sizes of pen cartridges—1.5 mL (150 units) and 3 mL (300 units).

Buying Insulin

Insulin is sold in any pharmacy and in most places it's available without a prescription. Each bottle or cartridge has an expiry date (usually one to two years after the purchase date). The insulin bottle should be discarded after that date.

Insulin costs roughly U.S. $20, or Cdn $20–$25, for 1,000 units. Insulin purchase is covered by some provincial government health care plans in Canada, and most insurance companies require a prescription in order to reimburse the cost.

Manufacturers of Insulin
Two manufacturers—Eli Lilly and Novo Nordisk Biochem—market insulin in North America. There is no difference in quality or selection of insulin products, with the exception of Lispro, which is currently available through Eli Lilly only. A list of available products is provided in the Further Resources section at the end of this book.

Care of Insulin
Insulin can be kept safely in the refrigerator until its expiry date. After it has been opened, it can be stored at room temperature for a month.

Insulin is a very stable substance that doesn't "go bad" easily. However, if it is allowed to freeze or get extremely hot, it can be damaged. Regular insulin that is cloudy or straw-colored instead of clear, or that has solid particles floating in it, should not be used. With NPH, Lente or Ultralente insulin, it is natural for the white substance to settle to the bottom of the bottle over a period of time. This should mix easily into the solution. Don't use cloudy insulin if particles or lumps are floating around after mixing, or if solid pieces stick to the bottom or side of the bottle. To be safe, if the insulin is exposed to an extreme temperature, discard the bottle. A new bottle should be started when there is less than about 10 percent of the insulin remaining in the old bottle.

If a child is hiking, camping or traveling long distances, protect bottles from breakage and temperature extremes by wrapping them individually and placing them in a small thermal container. Vigorous shaking—during horseback riding, for example—can make clear insulin turn cloudy. If this happens, discard the bottle. Always keep a spare bottle of insulin on hand in case one gets broken. For children using two kinds of insulin, keep a spare bottle of each type.

Injecting Insulin

Injecting a child with insulin is probably one of the biggest hurdles parents have to overcome. Many are squeamish about needles, never mind giving one to their own child. Teenagers, and indeed some younger children, quickly become quite adept at administering their own insulin. Initially, however, both parents need to become proficient too. Other caregivers such as grandparents and babysitters should also be able to give an injection in case of illness or emergency. Children who are preparing and injecting their own insulin must be supervised to ensure that the dose is accurate, the insulin is actually injected and the child doesn't favor the same injection site day after day. Supervision will remind them that insulin is important, and potentially dangerous if too much is given at one time. When both parents are involved, the mutual support encourages better family adaptation to diabetes.

Injecting with a Syringe and Needle

At first, parents and children learn to inject insulin with a syringe specifically designed to measure insulin. The syringe has three parts: the needle, the plunger and the barrel.

Insulin syringes are generally available in four sizes: 1/4 mL or 25 units, 3/10 mL or 30 units, 1/2 mL or 50 units, and 1 mL or 100 units. All are intended to measure 100 units per mL insulin, which is the standard strength available in North America. The larger the dose, the larger the syringe.

Syringes

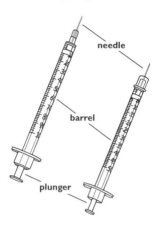

Needles are available in a variety of lengths and thicknesses, and are measured in gauges. The higher the gauge number, the finer the needle. The length of the needle varies from the standard half-inch (12.8 mm) to a newer, shorter 3/8-inch (8 mm) needle. Generally, children prefer finer needles because they hurt less. While shorter needles may be more comfortable for younger or thinner children, teenagers may choose longer needles to ensure the insulin is injected at the right depth.

Preparing a Single Type of Insulin

- Gather together the insulin, the syringe and needle and an alcohol swab. Wash your hands.
- Double-check the label on the insulin to make sure you have the right kind.
- Note the expiry date.
- If the insulin is NPH, Lente or Ultralente, roll the bottle gently four or five times between your hands to mix it thoroughly. Do not shake the bottle, or the insulin will become frothy and difficult to measure.

- Clean the top of the bottle with the alcohol swab and remove the cover from the needle.
- Pull back on the plunger to draw up air. You will need as many units of air as the units of insulin you will be injecting. If you are planning to inject 20 units of insulin, draw 20 units of air into the syringe.
- With the insulin bottle right side up, insert the needle into the rubber stopper on top of the bottle and push the plunger down so the air enters the top of the bottle. This equalizes the pressure and prevents a vacuum in the bottle, making it easier to withdraw the insulin. Avoid injecting air into the insulin itself.
- Leaving the needle in the bottle, turn the bottle upside down, making sure the tip of the needle is fully immersed in the insulin. Do not draw air into the syringe.
- Pull back the plunger to the number of units of insulin required. Ensure there are no air bubbles in the syringe, because they would take up space where insulin should be.
- Remove any air bubbles by flicking the syringe with your finger until they rise to the top. You may need to push the plunger upward to get rid of the air and then reset the plunger at the correct number of units. If the air is not removed, the dose will be inadequate.
- Double-check with another person that you have the correct kind and amount of insulin in the syringe, whenever possible.
- Take the needle out of the bottle and replace the cap if you are going to be moving to another room to do the injection. With younger children, these steps can be taken in a different room to create less disruption for the child.

Giving the Actual Injection
- Gather together the insulin-loaded syringe and a dry cotton swab or tissue.

- Select the injection site. (See illustration on page 43.)
- Gently pinch up the skin and fat with the thumb and fore-finger.
- Hold the syringe like a pencil, close to the needle for better control.
- Push the needle in quickly and all the way, at a 90-degree angle to the pinched-up skin.
- Push the plunger in to inject the insulin.
- Slowly let go of the pinched-up skin and then remove the needle.
- Using a dry swab, apply gentle pressure to the injection site to prevent bruising.
- Discard the needle and syringe in a special container, available at your pharmacy, or recycle a juice can or empty bleach container. To avoid possible injury, never leave used needles lying around.

Preparing a Mixture of Insulin Types

Most young people need two different types of insulin mixed in one injection. For instance, the pre-breakfast injection will likely include some fast-acting or superfast-acting insulin (Regular or Lispro) to work with the food in the coming meal, and some intermediate-acting insulin (NPH or Lente) that will peak later in the day.

Preparing an injection of two types of insulin is similar to preparing an injection of one type. The only difference is that you prepare both bottles of insulin (rolling, cleaning the tops and injecting the appropriate amounts of air) and then draw up the prescribed amounts from each bottle.

- Put as many units of air into the bottle of fast-acting (clear) insulin as you plan to draw out in insulin, but do not withdraw the insulin.
- Remove the needle from the clear insulin bottle, and put as

many units of air into the bottle of intermediate-acting (cloudy) insulin as you plan to draw out in insulin. Withdraw the prescribed amount of cloudy insulin.

- Make sure there are no large air bubbles.
- Now add the prescribed amount of fast-acting insulin to the same syringe.
- If you accidentally pull the plunger back too far when adding the second kind of insulin, discard the insulin in the syringe and begin again. If cloudy insulin is mixed into the clear insulin bottle by mistake, discard that bottle.
- Inject as usual.

You can also withdraw the fast-acting insulin first, followed by the intermediate-acting insulin.

Selecting the Injection Site
There are four safe areas for insulin injections.

- *Thighs:* top and outer areas only. Do not use the inner side or back of the thigh, and stay about four of the child's fingerwidths away from the knee and groin.
- *Upper arms:* fleshy area on the side and back of the arms. Avoid the muscle in the shoulder, and stay three to four fingerwidths away from the elbow.
- *Abdomen:* right across the abdomen, from just below the ribcage to well below the belt line. Stay about two fingerwidths away from the navel.
- *Buttocks:* fleshy area (i.e. jeans pocket area).

Insulin may be absorbed differently from one site than from another. Absorption is most predictable when injections are given in the abdomen and buttocks. In general, insulin injected into the upper arms or thighs is absorbed more erratically.

Also, insulin injected over an exercising muscle may be absorbed more quickly, so it's wise to avoid injecting into the arms or thighs of someone who's planning strenuous exercise including these muscles: i.e., runners should avoid injections into the thighs, rowers should avoid injections into the arms, and so on.

Injection sites

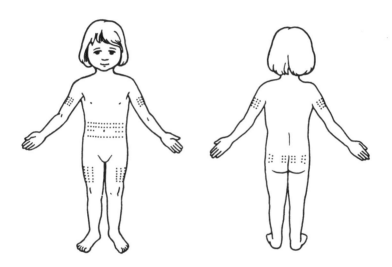

Injections are done in a pattern, to avoid using exactly the same site over and over. Ensure that each injection is about one inch (2.5 cm) or two fingerwidths from the previous one. Try to work in straight, even rows about an inch apart. This way you're more likely to remember where the last injection was given.

Rotating Injection Sites
Many people with diabetes, children especially, develop "favorite" injection sites where the pain seems to be less and

injections seem easier. If the same small area is used repeatedly, the fat tissue below the skin swells (*lipohypertrophy*). The swelling may produce large bumps that absorb insulin poorly. They may go away in time when the site is left alone. Until the lumps have disappeared, inject away from the lumps—not into them—to promote better insulin absorption. Sometimes repeated injections into the same site do not produce lipohypertrophy, but rather a hard area of scar tissue under the skin. These sites should also be avoided. At each clinic visit a member of the diabetes team will examine the injection areas to help with site selection and the prevention of lumps or bumps.

Injecting with Pens and Cartridges

A newer and sometimes more convenient method of injection is the insulin pen. Rather than withdrawing insulin from a bottle, you use a cartridge of insulin that fits into a pen-like device. A special needle-tip screws onto the end of the pen and, by adjusting the dial on the side of the pen, you can control the dose. You then push down on the end of the pen (like a plunger) and the insulin is delivered. Just as there are different sizes of insulin syringes, there are different-sized pens. One holds a cartridge of 150 units, the other a cartridge of 300 units. Manufacturers recommend changing the needle-tip after every use.

Needle-tips are available in the same gauges as the needles designed for syringes. However, because they don't have to go through the rubber stopper on the top of the insulin bottle, they may stay sharper and hurt less. They are also more discreet and quicker to prepare than a syringe. The main drawback is that you can't give two kinds of insulin in one injection. There are premixed insulin preparations that may be suitable for some children; however, you can't adjust the ratio of the mix. Insulin delivery by pens may also be a bit more expensive.

Other Devices

There are many devices designed to make injections seem easier; however, none takes away the need for an injection itself. Before investing in any injection aid, talk to your health care team about its usefulness and effectiveness. If your child wants an injection aid to eliminate pain, remind him that all injections hurt a little. If the injection is more painful than usual, try to:

- check the needle—there may be a defect
- insert the needle quickly—slow injections hurt more
- push the plunger in a little more slowly—this will reduce any burning sensation
- keep the insulin out of the refrigerator—children say they can feel cold insulin being injected
- pinch the skin less tightly
- try a different injection site

If none of this works, talk to your diabetes nurse about the selection of injection sites, different kinds of needles and other tools that may be helpful.

Insertion Aids

For those bothered by inserting a needle, these spring-loaded devices can be useful. With the push of a button, the needle of an insulin-filled syringe is quickly inserted under the skin. Generally, the plunger of the syringe must still be pushed to inject the insulin.

Jet Injectors

Jet injectors are needleless alternatives to syringes. They force insulin through the skin in a high-pressure stream. Although this may seem an ideal way of delivering insulin, injectors are very expensive and require consistent maintenance to keep them sterile. They can cause injury to the skin, such as bruising, and checking the accuracy of the dose can be difficult because some insulin may stay on the surface of the skin. They have not been shown to be less traumatic, physically or emotionally, to the child.

Insulin Pumps

Insulin pumps are about the size of a phone pager, and are worn on the belt or kept in a pocket. They deliver insulin continuously, through a small needle that remains under the skin. A catheter—a small plastic tube—connects the needle to the pump. The catheter and needle must be changed every few days. The pump holds a measured amount of insulin in a special syringe, and weighs less than four ounces (115 grams). The pump infuses a constant amount of insulin throughout the day and night (a *basal dose*). The user prompts a miniature computer to release a surge of insulin (a *bolus*) just before each meal to counter the effect of the food. The device beeps if the tube is clogged, if the batteries are running low or if too much insulin is being delivered. Users can change the rate of insulin according to their current needs—for example, during illness, when more insulin is required, or during periods of intense activity, when less insulin is required.

Pumps are very expensive, as much as $5,000 (both U.S. and Canadian), not including monthly costs for catheters and special syringes. Pumps are generally not appropriate for young children because they demand a great deal of time and attention, as well as blood checks four to seven times a day. A more appropriate candidate for an insulin pump would be the highly motivated teen who wants to maintain excellent control over blood sugar and is comfortable with technology, as well as with diabetes, given that the pump is somewhat obvious. Although it need not be conspicuous during most activities, it cannot always be hidden. A supportive family and a diabetes team familiar with pump treatment are also essential.

Insulin Dosages and Frequency

Initially, the health care team will determine the insulin dosage and frequency. This is the *insulin regimen*. It can take a few days to a few weeks of fine-tuning to figure out exactly how much insulin is required. In general, it is not possible to achieve and maintain excellent blood sugar control beyond the honeymoon period with one or two injections of intermediate-acting insulin alone. Eventually most children and teens need both fast-acting and intermediate-acting insulins, three or four times a day.

It is important to note that there are exceptions, but generally, to begin with, infants, toddlers and preschoolers receive two injections a day: a mixture of fast-acting or superfast-acting and intermediate-acting insulins before breakfast and again before supper.

Older children (over five or six years of age) and teens usually start on three injections a day, using a mix of fast-acting or superfast-acting and intermediate-acting insulin before breakfast, fast-acting or superfast-acting insulin before supper and intermediate-acting insulin at bedtime. Some centers prescribe insulin twice daily to start, combining the fast-acting and intermediate-acting at suppertime.

Some older teens prefer to move to, or even start on, a four-injection-a-day routine, with a dose of superfast-acting or fast-acting insulin before breakfast, lunch and supper, and intermediate-acting insulin at bedtime.

Since insulin requirements are affected by growth and

development, appetite, physical activity and stress or illness, no fixed dose will work indefinitely. The dose must be adjusted to provide optimal blood glucose control.

In time, as blood glucose levels stabilize and families gain more experience, most parents and teens become quite adept at taking the lead in decisions about adjustments. The diabetes team is always there for advice and backup.

Q&A

I hate needles. How can I expect my six-year-old to get used to them?

Children take their cues from their parents. Any fear or dislike you have of needles may make your child afraid too. Some parents find that reminding themselves that the insulin injection allows their child to survive and stay healthy makes injection time easier. If parents say, "I need to give you your insulin so you'll have lots of energy to play and to grow," the child begins to understand, and the parents get over their own apprehension. Follow up each needle with a big hug and kiss, and get on with the day's activities.

My toddler gets a combination of NPH and Regular insulin twice each day. Because the dose is so tiny, it seems I discard the better part of both 10 mL bottles of insulin at the end of each month. Is there any reason I can't use a syringe to withdraw the insulin from a cartridge instead?

Although the insulin manufacturers don't suggest substituting cartridges for bottles, many people find that if they need less than 10 or 15 units of NPH or Regular or Lispro insulin it's less costly to use pen cartridges (either the 1.5 mL or the 3.0 mL) in place of 10 mL bottles. The unopened cartridges can be stored in the refrigerator until the expiry date, and the open cartridge is discarded after four weeks. If you choose to substitute cartridges for bottles of insulin, there are some important differences in technique.

Don't attempt to put any air into the cartridge before withdrawing the insulin. Simply insert the needle and withdraw the insulin. Inserting air is not only unnecessary but may result in popping out the cork at the other end of the cartridge, in which case the entire cartridge will be ruined.

Also, in preparing NPH insulin you'll need to shake the cartridge up and down 10 times. As you do this, you'll see a glass bead moving up and down, mixing the insulin. Rolling the cartridge between your hands doesn't work, because there is no air in the cartridge to allow the insulin solution to move around and mix evenly.

Our five-year-old prefers that Mommy give the injections. Is that a problem?
In many families, one person takes on most of the responsibility for injections. Problems arise, however, when that person is unavailable. It's important that all regular caregivers be able to share responsibility for giving the injection, and that the child feel safe and confident with any of them. Single-parent families should enlist the help of a friend or relative. Some families work out a schedule where one parent takes care of the morning injections and the other parent looks after evening injections.

Sharing the burden is also critical for coping with the daily demands of diabetes and preventing parent burnout.

How old do children have to be before they can give their own injections?
There's no magic age at which children are suddenly capable. Generally, by nine or ten years of age, they have the manual

dexterity and ability to draw up and give their own insulin. However, children this age lack judgment. They may not take great care drawing up the exact dose. Or, if they forget to give themselves an injection before school, they may not realize the importance of returning home for it. Young people usually require supervision into their teenage years. This means watching your child prepare the dose and insert the needle, checking the expiry date on the insulin bottle and reminding the child to rotate injection sites.

Even at younger ages, many children are curious and want to take part in some aspects of the routine. As they reach the age when they want to go on sleepovers or spend more time away from home, it will become more important for them to show that they can safely manage their own diabetes routines. This is a gradual process for both parents and child. Many children learn to give their first needle or to try new sites at diabetes summer camps.

Sometimes the needle seems to get clogged. What should I do?
The needle can sometimes become clogged with cloudy insulin, usually after some of the insulin has been injected. The problem is, how much clear insulin and how much cloudy insulin has gone in? Remove the needle, noting how much insulin remains. If you're using a mixture of clear and cloudy insulin, prepare the full dose of insulin again, squirt out (waste) the amount that's already been injected, and inject the remaining insulin.

What if some insulin leaks out of the injection site?
Sometimes this just happens. When insulin does leak, *don't* try to guess the amount lost and replace it. The risk of too much insulin causing a low blood sugar reaction outweighs any

benefit. Note it in your logbook and take it into account if the next blood check is high. In the meantime, here are a few tips to minimize such occurrences:

- Get rid of any cause of excess pressure at the injection site, such as a bent leg or a chair pressing against the buttock.
- Gently pinch the skin and pull it slightly to the side before injecting. When you let go, the skin falls back into place and covers the needle track.
- Inject the insulin slowly.
- Let go of the pinched skin before removing the needle to avoid squeezing the insulin back out.
- Count to five before removing the needle.
- Apply light pressure on the injection site for a couple of seconds as you remove the needle, to prevent blood and insulin from coming out.

What does it mean if there is bruising at the injection site?
This can happen from time to time and it's not harmful. It usually means the needle has nicked a tiny blood vessel. To minimize the chance of bruising, apply gentle pressure to the site with a dry piece of cotton or a clean finger after injecting. Also, be careful not to pinch the skin too tightly or insert the needle too slowly. If you get continuous and excessive bruising, consult your doctor.

Are premixed insulins better than mixing your own insulin?
Not necessarily. Premixed insulins may be more convenient, but they don't give you as much flexibility. With children, the insulin dose changes frequently due to growth and varying appetite and activity. Ideally, families should be able to alter doses of intermediate and fast-acting insulins, independent of each other. Premixes don't allow for this.

Some of my son's friends clean their injection sites with alcohol.
But my son refuses to. Should I be worried?
There are more important things to worry about. In fact, most diabetes centers no longer include alcohol swabbing as part of their injection technique. There's no evidence to show that brief alcohol swabbing has any effect when people bathe regularly. Injection-site infections are exceptionally rare.

Why is the injection site all red and itchy?
Some children are sensitive to rubbing alcohol or one of the components of the insulin solution. The redness you see is probably a hive—a localized allergic reaction. Changing the brand of insulin may help, or switching from NPH to Lente (or vice versa). But the redness will likely go away on its own. In rare cases, someone has an allergic reaction to insulin. Speak to your diabetes team. In most cases the child eventually builds up a tolerance to the insulin and the reaction subsides.

What happens if you accidentally give too much insulin?
Believe it or not, this is not an uncommon mistake. If you've given too much insulin, contact your health care team. You'll need to monitor blood sugar levels every two to three hours. Set your alarm to wake you up through the night if necessary. You will need to provide extra food to help keep the blood sugar level up to balance the high insulin level.

What would happen if I accidentally injected an air bubble into my child?
Everyone worries about the risk of injecting an air bubble. It's not harmful to inject an air bubble under the skin, but if you're injecting air rather than insulin, your child may not be getting the full dose. This will cause a high blood sugar reading.

F O U R

Making Meals Work

ealtime at Terry and Linda's home is always lively. Both parents like to prepare interesting dishes for their two sons, Michael, 12, and Campbell, 8, who has diabetes. The family's diet is healthy, featuring a variety of foods, even though vegetables are not a favorite. Before being diagnosed with diabetes, Campbell didn't have much of a sweet tooth. However, like most children, he did enjoy the occasional treat.

"I remember when Campbell was diagnosed," recalls Linda. "It was just before his fifth birthday. I was so worried that he wouldn't be allowed to eat any sugar. How were we going to celebrate his birthday without cake and ice cream?" After speaking to the dietitian in the hospital, Linda realized that they didn't have to make many changes in their eating habits, and that with some planning Campbell could have the cake and ice cream on his birthday.

Even though Campbell has had diabetes for three and a half years, Linda and Terry still sometimes find meal planning a challenge. "This winter was Campbell's first year playing hockey," says Terry, noting that early morning practices, suppertime games and weekend tournaments present a change from his usual eating routines. But with careful planning, they were able to make the necessary adjustments.

For some families, planning meals is the trickiest part of diabetes management. At first, you look at food very differently than you did before. The simple act of cooking dinner can feel like a science class, with all the weights and measures. The grocery shopping trips often take much longer than in the past, as nutrition information on food labels gains importance.

What Is a Diabetes Meal Plan?

Because children with diabetes lack automatic blood sugar regulation—they can't "turn off" the injected insulin—a steady supply of glucose, in the form of carbohydrate, must be provided to maintain their blood glucose balance and avoid excessive lows and highs. A meal plan consists of three main meals and one to three snacks each day. The goal is to have a consistent amount of carbohydrate at the same time each day, to make it easier to determine the appropriate insulin dose. It's important that the amount of food satisfy the appetite and provide enough nutrients for proper growth. *Consistency* is key to a successful meal plan. However, any meal plan must be flexible and realistic, and

---

The main goals of the meal plan

- to satisfy appetite
- to promote normal growth and development
- to balance sugar
- to be easy to follow so the family can incorporate it into their daily lives

must take into account the individual's lifestyle, likes and dislikes.

How Foods Affect Blood Sugar

Ask people what they know about diabetes, and chances are they'll say, "That's the disease where you can't eat sugar, right?" In fact, people with diabetes can and do eat sugar. The catch is that they have to pay closer attention to what kinds of sugar they eat, how much they eat and when they eat it. Many foods contain some form of sugar; learning how much sugar different foods contain is an important aspect of diabetes nutrition.

The foods we eat provide many nutrients, which are divided into three main food groups or *macronutrients*: protein, fat and carbohydrate. (Vitamins and minerals are *micronutrients*.) Many foods are a combination of protein, fat and carbohydrate, and therefore appear in all three categories in the food list below.

Carbohydrates
- *Starches:* breads, pasta, rice, grains, cereals, corn, potatoes, cookies, crackers
- *Fruit and vegetables:* all fruits and fruit juices, including tomato juice; vegetables that have a sweetish taste, such as turnip, squash, carrots, peas, beets, parsnip
- *Dairy products:* milk, yogurt, ice cream
- *Sugars:* refined sugar, honey, molasses, syrups; jams and jellies; candy; chocolate; regular soft drinks

It's important to consider carbohydrates, or sugars, in diabetes meal plans because this is the only group that directly and immediately raises blood sugar levels. As you can see above, carbohydrates are found in a variety of foods, from grains (breads, pasta) and fruits to milk and chocolate. Carbohydrates are an essential source of energy.

There are two types of carbohydrates—simple and complex. *Simple carbohydrates* are made up of single or paired sugar molecules that are rapidly broken down by the body to provide a quick source of sugar. They include *fructose* (found in fruits and vegetables), *sucrose* (found in refined sugar products) and *lactose* (found in dairy products). When you are reading ingredients labels, note that words ending in *ose* can be classified as sugars. For example, *dextrose* and *maltose* are both sugars. Honey, corn syrup and liquid invert sugar are other common sweeteners that contain simple carbohydrates and raise blood glucose levels. Artificial sweeteners (such as sucralose, saccharin and aspartame) do not.

People with diabetes can eat sugar and foods containing added sugar, such as candy and chocolate, in moderation—up to 10 percent of their total calorie intake. Learning how to incorporate such foods into the diet makes the meal plan easier to follow.

Complex carbohydrates, on the other hand, take longer for the body to digest. Therefore these foods take longer to turn into energy than simple carbohydrates. Complex carbohydrates are found in starch-based foods.

Protein
- Meat, poultry, fish, shellfish
- Eggs
- Legumes (nuts, beans and lentils, peanuts and peanut butter, tofu)
- Milk, cheese, cottage cheese and other dairy products

With the exception of milk, yogurt, ice cream and legumes (which also contain carbohydrate), protein foods do not directly raise blood glucose levels. (During prolonged starvation or undernutrition the body can break them down into sugar.) Proteins are essential for growth and to promote healing and tissue repair. Protein foods also provide essential vitamins and minerals.

Fats

- *All oils:* lard, shortening, margarine
- *Meat:* especially red meat, but also fowl
- *Fish and shellfish*
- *Dairy products:* butter, milk, cream and cream products, cheese and cheese products
- *Eggs*
- *Other:* salad dressings (low fat and regular), gravies, nuts, seeds, olives, coconut, avocado

Fats are the major component of such foods as butter, margarine, oil, most salad dressings and gravies. Fats are an important part of a well-balanced diet because they also provide essential building blocks for growth and development.

There are three types of fats.

- *Saturated fats* are usually solid at room temperature and tend to raise blood cholesterol. They are found in lard, shortening, butter, and animal products such as meat, eggs and milk.
- *Polyunsaturated fats*, which are found in vegetable oils such as safflower, sunflower, corn and soybean, sesame and most nut oils, are usually liquid at room temperature. Nuts and seeds, or soft margarines made with these oils, tend to be associated with lower blood cholesterol.
- *Monounsaturated fats* are found in other oils, including olive, peanut and canola, as well as soft margarine made from these oils. These fats may lower blood cholesterol levels if used in place of saturated fats.

These three types of fats are found in varying combinations in foods. It is wise to try to limit the amount of fat in the diet, and to try to choose foods that contain polyunsaturated or monounsaturated fats. Maintaining normal lipid (blood fat) levels is important, as high levels contribute to the risk of developing certain complications later in life.

Some vegetables—lettuce, celery, cucumbers and peppers, for example—fall outside the three categories of carbohydrates, proteins and fats. They are essential, however, because they add vitamins, minerals and fiber to the diet, as well as flavor and variety. Since they don't contain macronutrients, they can be considered "free" foods.

Meal Planning for the Infant or Toddler

Infants and toddlers experience daily fluctuations in appetite, making it difficult to stick to a meal plan. One day they may have a spoonful of cereal for breakfast, nibble at a sandwich for lunch and have a tiny piece of meat for supper. The next day it may be an entire bowl of cereal to start the day, milk and cookies for snacks, a peanut butter sandwich and banana for lunch and chicken and potatoes for supper. Young children may go through periods when they want to eat the same thing every day, followed by periods when they refuse to touch their previous favorites.

It is neither practical nor realistic to set up a strict meal plan for a young child with diabetes. Rather, meal planning should focus on normal infant or toddler feeding, emphasizing consistency in the timing of meals and snacks and avoiding an excessive amount of simple sugars such as juices. As children grow older, this approach can be changed to incorporate the principles of meal planning outlined below. This often occurs when the child starts spending more time in a school setting, such as the transition from kindergarten to first grade. In the meantime, it may be helpful to learn the carbohydrate content of different foods (see Carbohydrate Counting, later in this chapter), to offer a consistent amount of carbohydrate from day to day.

Setting Up the Meal Plan

The meal plan provides the framework for healthy eating and safe blood sugar control. Regular mealtimes and snack times and consistent amounts of food are key elements of the plan. *All* children with diabetes require three regular meals and a bedtime snack every day, to avoid low blood sugar emergencies. For most children the meal plan also includes a mid-afternoon snack. Some children, especially younger ones, have a regular mid-morning snack as well. How is the meal plan developed? How do you know the timing of meals and snacks, and how much food to offer? These are important questions.

A registered dietitian (RD) who is experienced in nutrition planning for children and adolescents and is a member of the diabetes team will help develop a meal plan to meet the needs of this particular child and family. The meal plan is based on what and how much food is normally eaten. Food intake records are important in helping the dietitian determine the initial food requirement, as well as changes down the line. The family records the amount and types of food eaten at each meal and snack over a period of about three days. The dietitian reviews these records and calculates the average amount of carbohydrate, protein and fat eaten at each meal and snack. This forms the basis of an "exchange-type" diet. The timing of meals and snacks depends on the family's routines. As the child grows and daily routines change, the meal plan must be altered to reflect these changes.

An alternative to this plan is to focus only on the carbohydrate content of each meal. This "carbohydrate counting" is a more flexible approach to meal planning, and may be most appropriate for older teens and adults who can apply the principles they have learned.

Each of these meal planning strategies requires careful attention to eating a specific amount of carbohydrate at each meal and snack.

The "Food Choice" or Exchange System

The Canadian Diabetes Association choice system organizes food into seven groups, based on protein, fat and carbohydrate content. Carbohydrates are further divided into starches (grains and cereals), fruits, vegetables, dairy products and sugars.

The American Diabetes Association exchange system is similar in principle to the Canadian system but organizes foods into six rather than seven groups including bread/starch, meat/protein, milk, fruit, vegetable and fat. It is worth noting that the carbohydrate content in some of the food groups is different in the Canadian and American exchange lists. The following table compares the grams of carbohydrate content in each system.

Exchange group	Canadian system	American system
bread/starch	15 grams	15 grams
fruit	10 grams	15 grams
vegetable	10 grams	5 grams
sugars	10 grams	——
meat/protein	0 grams	0 grams
fat	0 grams	0 grams
milk	4 oz = 6 grams	8 oz = 12 grams
(1 exchange)		

Sample exchanges or choices

(Each food item reflects one choice from that group)

Starch—15 gm carb.

- 1 slice bread
- 1/2 cup (125 mL) unsweetened cereal
- 1/2 hamburger bun or hotdog bun
- 3 cups (700 mL) popped popcorn
- 1/2 cup (125 mL) cooked rice
- 1/2 cup (125 mL) kernel corn (frozen or canned with no sugar added) or half a cob
- 2 cookies
- 1 small plain roll
- 1/2 cup cooked spaghetti
- 8 soda crackers
- 1 cup (250 mL) canned soup

Fruit and veg—10 gm carb.

- 1/2 medium apple
- 1/2 banana
- 1/2 cup (125 mL) blueberries
- 1 cup (250 mL) watermelon
- 1/2 cup (125 mL) carrots
- 1/2 cup (125 mL) beets
- 1 orange
- 1 cup (250 mL) strawberries

Milk—6 gm carb.

- 1/2 cup (125 mL) milk
- 1/2 cup (125 mL) yogurt

Sugars—10 gm carb.

- 2 tsp (10 mL) sugar
- 4 jelly beans
- 2 marshmallows

Fat choices

- 1 tsp (5 mL) butter, margarine or oil
- 1 slice bacon
- 1 tbsp (15 mL) cheese spread
- 1 tbsp (15 mL) cream cheese
- 1 tbsp (15 mL) salad dressing

Protein choices

- 1 oz (30 gm) cheese
- 1 oz (30 gm) ground meat
- 4 tbsp (60 mL) canned fish

Extras

- diet pop
- broccoli
- cucumber
- celery
- green pepper

Based on the food records, the dietitian plans a certain number of choices from each group for the child's meals and snacks. The number of carbohydrates per exchange is based on the amount in an average serving. This exchange system will become easy to apply, with some instruction from your dietitian and some practice using available lists.

Pino is 12 years old. Now that his normal appetite has returned, the dietitian has provided him and his parents with a meal plan. Here's a look at how many portions of each group Pino eats during the day:

	Breakfast	Snack	Lunch	Snack	Supper	Snack
	8:00 a.m.	10:00 a.m.	12:00	3:00 p.m.	6:00 p.m.	9:00 p.m.
starch	2	1	3	1	4	2
fruit & veg	2		2	2	1	2
milk (skim)	2		2		2	
protein	1		2		2	1
fat	2	1	2	1	2	2
extras			yes		yes	

Pino's meal plan calls for a supper consisting of 4 starch choices, 1 fruit and vegetable choice, 2 milk choices, 2 protein choices and 2 fat choices. Tonight the family is having spaghetti and meat sauce, salad, rolls and, for dessert, strawberries. So Pino can have:

4 starches • 2 cups (454 gm) spaghetti or 1 1/2 cups (340 gm) spaghetti plus a small dinner roll

1 fruit & veg • 1 cup (250 mL) strawberries

2 milks • 1 cup (250 mL) milk

2 proteins	• 2 oz (60 gm) ground meat (in meat sauce)
2 fats	• 2 tbsp (30 mL) salad dressing
Extras	• salad with lettuce, celery, peppers

Remember that a meal plan is not a diet in the sense of limiting food. It's important for Pino to feel satisfied, so his meal plan will change as he grows. He and his parents need to be aware when he starts to feel hungrier. Then the dietitian will help them adjust the meal plan to allow more food, and the doctor or diabetes nurse will adjust his insulin dosage to balance the effect of the extra food on his blood sugar.

Carbohydrate Counting
This approach to meal planning considers only the total amount of carbohydrate taken at each meal and snack. The amount of carbohydrate eaten, not the source, is what matters. After a careful assessment, the dietitian will recommend how much carbohydrate the child should eat each time.

Food group	*Grams of carbohydrate per choice*
starch	15 gm
fruit & veg	10 gm
milk	6 gm
sugars	10 gm

For example, a standard breakfast might include:

• 2 starch	2 x 15 g = 30 gm
• 2 fruit	2 x 10 g = 20 gm
• 2 milk	2 x 6 g = 12 gm
Total	62 gm

The child therefore needs about 62 grams of carbohydrate at breakfast. The same method can be used for other meals and snacks.

Sarah has had diabetes for two years. At age 14 she finds there are many different foods she wants to try, but she isn't sure how to work them into her meal plan. Also, the milk she brings to school for lunch is becoming an inconvenience, but she loves milk at home. The dietitian suggests carbohydrate counting to increase Sarah's flexibility.

Sarah's meal plan for lunch is:

- 3 starches
- 1 fruit
- 2 milk
- 2 protein
- 2 fat

She usually takes one sandwich, two cookies, 1/2 cup (125 mL) grapes or equivalent fruit and 1 cup (250 mL) of milk.

The dietitian uses the grams of carbohydrate per choice to determine that Sarah eats 67 grams of carbohydrate at lunch.

• 3 starch	3 x 15 gm = 45 gm	
• 1 fruit	1 x 10 gm = 10 gm	
• 2 milk	2 x 6 gm = 12 gm	
Total	67 gm	

Sarah needs to be within plus or minus 3 grams of 67 grams every day at lunch. Now on schooldays she eats different lunches. Friday she took:

- 1 hamburger bun with   30 gm (only the bun counts)
  roast beef, lettuce,
  tomato and mayonnaise
- 2 cookies   15 gm
- 1 apple   20 gm
- <u>1 diet iced tea</u>   <u>0 gm</u>
Total   65 gm (±3 gm)

At home on Saturday she ate:

- salad   0 gm
- 1 cup mushroom soup   15 gm
- 1 bagel   30 gm
- 1 cup milk   12 gm
- <u>1 cup strawberries</u>   <u>10 gm</u>
Total   67 gm

By eliminating milk from her weekday lunches, Sarah can have more variety and flexibility at school.

The Importance of Consistency

To achieve and maintain the best possible blood glucose control, all children and teens should try to be consistent from day to day in the timing, amount and types of foods eaten at meals and snacks. If, for example, a 12-year-old boy eats an enormous dinner one night but skips dinner the next, it makes the task of adjusting his insulin dose and preventing high and low blood sugar reactions very difficult. Some older teens and adults learn to use a different dose of fast-acting insulin before meals to allow for some flexibility and spontaneity. This will be discussed in the next chapter.

Knowing that mealtimes and the amounts of food eaten are consistent also helps rule out food as the cause of high or low blood sugar readings. For example, a new after-school activity is planned. The extra exercise will likely cause a lower blood sugar reading. If the child has swayed from the meal plan, and perhaps skipped a snack too, the parents can't be sure of the real cause of the low blood sugar.

Joey arrives home from school earlier than expected because his soccer practice is canceled. He usually has his snack before practice at 3:30 p.m., but since he doesn't have practice today, and he's not really that hungry, he decides to skip it. By 4:00 p.m., however, he is feeling hungry, so he eats his snack then. When he checks his blood sugar at 5:30 p.m., it's a little high. Is it high because he didn't burn off the energy he usually does during soccer practice, or because he had his snack later than usual and didn't have two hours between eating and testing his blood sugar? Because he was inconsistent in the timing of his afternoon snack, it is harder to determine the cause of the high sugar reading.

While not every high or low blood sugar reading can or should be accounted for, understanding the relationships between food, insulin and activity is important to help you determine whether an insulin adjustment is necessary. It's tempting to try to correct high or low readings by overeating or withholding food, but this can lead to a lot of confusion. For example, let's look at Joey again. His 5:30 p.m. reading is high, so he eats less dinner in order to bring down his blood glucose level. Before bed, he's a little low so he eats a few extra cookies. He gets up twice that night to go to the bathroom and wakes up with a high reading. To avoid increasing his blood sugar

---

Fast food

Diabetes doesn't mean that families can no longer enjoy the convenience of "fast food." Here are some exchange guidelines for common fast food fare:

- 1 hamburger = 2 starch, 2 protein, 2 fat
- 1 small fries (about 20) = 2 starch, 2 fat
- 1 slice medium cheese pizza = 2 starch, 2 protein, 2 fat
- 6-inch (15 cm) submarine sandwich = 3 starch, 2 protein, 2 fat

Most fast-food chains can supply exchange guidelines for their menus, on request.

---

further, he has half a bowl of cereal instead of a whole bowlful. By morning recess he starts to feel faint and nauseated with a low blood sugar reaction. This roller coaster is known as "chasing blood sugars." It can be frustrating and potentially dangerous.

Eating Out

For the first few weeks after diagnosis, parents may be nervous about taking their child out for dinner. But they shouldn't feel shy about explaining to waiters that someone in the family has diabetes and that, if the meal will be delayed, they need to know. In this event, nibbling on a breadstick or some crackers until the meal arrives is a good strategy, but these should be included as exchanges or part of the meal's carbohydrates.

Friends who don't know much about diabetes may be worried about what to feed the child. It helps to take the lead and invite friends over first so they can see that Joey still eats hotdogs, just as he used to. When eating at a friend's house, ask what time they intend to serve dinner and provide some guidance. Children may be able to switch their bedtime snack and dinner if dinner is being served much later than usual.

Q&A

Can my child have birthday cake again?
Yes. In fact, many children are so excited with the fun and games of the party that the food stays on the plate. The key is to ensure that the adult in charge is aware that the child needs to eat something. If the cake is loaded with icing, encourage the child to leave some icing on the plate. And if the blood sugar is high that evening, note the reason in your child's logbook, and move on.

What about Hallowe'en?
Hallowe'en is a special time of year for many children and parents alike. Children with diabetes shouldn't be deprived of the chance to dress up and parade around the neighborhood in search of treats. However, the treats should be monitored and should be worked into the meal plan. Remember that Hallowe'en night's extra activity should be planned for with extra food—perhaps one small chocolate bar for each 20 to 30 minutes out on the streets. The remaining treats can be part of a meal or snack or can be used as extra food for planned activities. Remember how you handled Hallowe'en candy before your child had diabetes, and try not to make too much of it. Trade some of the lollipops, candy and regular gum for chips, sugarless gum or even a trip to the movies. Be creative!

People keep telling me that lentils and beans are good for people with diabetes. Should I introduce these into my family's diet?
Lentils and beans are excellent sources of low-fat protein and are commonly suggested for people with Type 2 diabetes. If you already prepare dishes using these foods, that's fine. Do not feel, however, that you should make radical changes in the foods your family eats. Adjusting to diabetes is difficult enough! If you want to introduce new foods to your table, wait

until you have the other aspects of diabetes management—blood glucose testing, insulin injections and the meal plan—under control. Some legumes produce bloating and gas, so go slowly if these are not a usual part of your family's diet.

My three-year-old only wants to eat macaroni. Is this normal?
Many younger children have a limited number of foods they like to eat. However, children—especially toddlers—will decide on a whim that what was the only food choice for three weeks is now totally unacceptable. With a child with diabetes, be ready to offer other appealing options. Foods such as cereal or a grilled cheese sandwich are good choices. Keep food fun by arranging servings in a unique way, or cutting food into interesting shapes. Children love to dip anything—vegetables into dip, crackers into soup. They may also respond to food more readily if they are involved in choosing it. Ask what they want from the grocery store, or have them help fill the cart. You can even involve them in preparing the dish in a safe, appropriate way, such as arranging chopped vegetables in a dish.

My toddler sometimes decides he doesn't want to eat—after I've already given the insulin. Should I force him to eat?
Forcing a child to eat usually leaves both the parents and the child upset and frustrated. Toddlers will usually take juice or milk, both sources of carbohydrate. Watch carefully for a low blood sugar reaction and treat it appropriately. They'll probably be hungry for their next meal or snack, since they ate little or nothing earlier. If food refusal happens often, talk to your diabetes team. You may need to reduce the insulin and adjust the blood sugar targets. Or ask your doctor about giving the insulin injection immediately after the meal. This may work best with superfast-acting insulin (Lispro).

Is it safe to eat a vegetarian diet with diabetes?
A vegetarian diet is safe for people with diabetes, provided all nutritional needs are being met, as in people without diabetes. Your dietitian will be a great source of information and support as you strive to make healthy choices.

What about fasting—can people with diabetes participate in rituals of Ramadan or Yom Kippur?
Fasting is extremely risky for anyone who takes insulin. Generally, people with diabetes are exempt from these rituals, but check with the appropriate religious authority. In many cases, specific guidelines have been worked out.

Do I really need to start weighing and measuring all these portions?
It may seem inconvenient at first, but weighing and measuring food will help you learn to estimate what a portion size is. After a while, you won't need to double-check every measurement. However, it's a good idea to go back to weighing and measuring foods from time to time, to be sure that your estimates are still fairly accurate.

I'm going crazy counting carbohydrates. I'm worried about making a mistake.
Initially, many parents are overwhelmed by the amount of planning and measuring involved in following a meal plan, and start to plan their meals according to the number of carbohydrates suggested. Instead, it's easier to plan meals as you usually would, and then look at the carbohydrate count and give appropriate portions. Remember to include food from all food groups—grains and cereals, fruits and vegetables, meats and

alternates and dairy products—and you'll be providing a balanced diet that meets the requirements of diabetes.

Should I put my child on a low-fat diet, or can we still eat burgers and fries occasionally?

Fat is an important part of a growing child's diet, and you should resist eliminating it from the diet altogether. However, we don't generally have to go out of our way to work fat into the North American child's diet. The occasional meal of burgers and fries can be part of a healthy diet.

My child puts ketchup on everything. Is the sugar in ketchup going to affect his blood sugar?

The small amount of sugar (3 grams or less in 2 tsp/10 mL) found in *reasonable* serving sizes of ketchup, barbecue sauce, store-bought salad dressings or peanut butter is not enough to elevate blood sugar levels significantly.

Is it safe to use sugar substitutes?

The sweeteners commonly found in grocery stores, which are also in diet foods and diet drinks, have been approved by the government. For most of these products the government has set an acceptable daily intake (ADI), which is the average amount people can use every day of their lives without risk of harm. The ADI is based on body weight, but there's a very large safety margin. The dietitian on your team can give you specific information about particular sweeteners.

It's worth noting that some sweeteners, such as sorbitol (often found in gum and dietetic candy), can have a slight laxative effect.

FIVE

Balancing Blood Sugar

ason, 12, isn't very athletic, but he loves a snowy winter
evening—especially when it's not a school night. Often,
on a Friday night after dinner, he and his friends head
off to the local toboggan hill for a couple of hours of slipping
and sliding. Jason has diabetes, but he has no trouble keeping
up with his tobogganing buddies. He can easily match them
run for run. In fact, he can even join them for a nice big mug
of hot chocolate with marshmallows at the end of the evening.
Jason has learned he can do almost anything his friends can
do, with a little planning.

Jason knows that walking up the toboggan hill will use
up a lot of energy. If he takes his usual amount of insulin
and eats the usual amount of food, his blood sugar will go
low—probably when he's out on the hill. He also knows that
he can't pass up the hot chocolate on these nights—after all,
tobogganing and hot chocolate go hand in hand. So he and
his parents agree on a slight reduction in the suppertime
fast-acting insulin, a mug of hot chocolate after tobogganing, and a blood sugar test before bed. Even though hot

chocolate is a higher-sugar bedtime snack than usual, the extra activity after dinner means Jason can afford the extra carbohydrate.

As parents and child or teen continue to learn more about diabetes, they begin to feel more confident about the decisions they are making. Children become accustomed to checking their blood sugar level three or four times a day; parents are less nervous about giving insulin injections; older children start to recognize the feelings they get when their blood glucose starts to fall. Parents consult their diabetes team less often, primarily because they now know the answers to a lot of their own questions and are better able to deal with new situations. By including children in the discussion and problem-solving, they can pave the way for future independence.

Blood sugar monitoring is essential in evaluating the blood sugar balance and diabetes control. Other tools include urine testing for sugar and ketones, and a blood test for hemoglobin A_{1c} or glycosylated hemoglobin, which reflects diabetes control over a three-month period.

You should become familiar with these tools. Such checks are useful only when they are done accurately and interpreted wisely.

Setting the Blood Glucose Target Range

The blood sugar targets change at various stages of growth and development. Target ranges are defined by the child's and parents' or other caregiver's ability to understand diabetes, interpret signs and feelings of low blood sugar levels, and act on them. They are negotiated with the diabetes team, all of whom should have the same goals.

Blood glucose target ranges

Age	Characteristic/ability	Acceptable target range (before meals)
infants/toddlers/ preschoolers	• unable to recognize or communicate signs and symptoms of low blood sugar reaction • unpredictable eating	6–12 mmol/L (110–220 mg/dL)
school-age children and some young adolescents	• more predictable eating (meal plan) • able to recognize and communicate symptoms of low blood sugar reaction • somewhat lacking in judgment • reliant on others for adjusting treatment and planning ahead	4–10 mmol/L (70–180 mg/dL)
most adolescents and young adults	• capable of predictable eating • able to recognize and treat low blood sugar reactions • understand concept of balance • able to plan ahead	4–8 mmol/L (70–145 mg/dL) —range may be different for those on intensive management

When to Check Blood Glucose

Checking blood glucose levels before each meal and before the bedtime snack tells you how the daily insulin is working. But one test cannot tell the whole story. Each test gives a unique and important piece of information. For example, the pre-breakfast test tells you how well the dinner or bedtime intermediate-acting insulin worked during the night; the pre-lunch and pre-supper tests tell you (respectively) how well the fast-acting and intermediate-acting insulin taken at breakfast are working, or how the fast-acting insulin taken at lunch is working; the pre-bedtime test provides information about the fast-acting insulin taken at supper.

In general, testing before meals provides more useful information than testing after meals, when levels will be predictably higher, providing an inaccurate picture of glucose balance. If insulin is increased on the basis of these "false high" readings, the blood sugar may go too low at other times.

Glucose testing four times a day (before each meal and before the bedtime snack) is ideal but may not be practical. For example, a lunchtime check in young children in daycare or school may be difficult. But a minimum of three tests should be done each day: one before breakfast and the others before the evening meal and the bedtime snack. An occasional check in the middle of the night helps detect those at risk for late-night lows.

Sometimes blood sugar should be checked apart from the routine—for example, before, during or after a vigorous activity such as a dance class or football practice, to determine how that particular activity affects the child's glucose level, or during illness or other times of stress.

If the blood sugar is consistently outside the target range (too low or too high), at least four daily checks are needed to determine the appropriate insulin dose adjustment. It is also useful to check between midnight and four a.m., as this is often the lowest time of the day.

Additional testing should also be done:
- if symptoms of low blood sugar are present
- every four hours during an illness
- at other times prescribed by the doctor, or when you're trying to problem-solve or gather information about the impact of a certain food or activity

How to Check Blood Glucose

Since about 1980 it has been possible for people with diabetes to check their blood sugar levels at home. While home blood sugar monitoring may not be quite as precise as laboratory methods, it is certainly accurate enough for daily assessment of diabetes control. There are two methods for home checking—visually, or with a blood glucose meter. Both methods require a drop of blood from a finger prick.

The blood sample is placed on or in a small area on a special test strip. With visual strips and some meter strips a color change occurs. With other meters an electrical current is activated. In all cases, the reaction depends on the blood sugar level.

Lancing device and meter

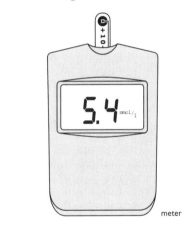

meter

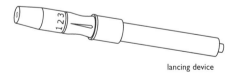

lancing device

Today, most families choose to buy a blood glucose meter. This provides accurate, quick readings of blood glucose when

used correctly. Visual strips may be useful as a back-up in case of meter failure; you compare the color to a chart on the side of the box.

Lancing devices are tools that, at the touch of a button, activate a *lancet* to prick the finger to obtain a drop of blood. The actual lancet is a small plastic insert with a very short needle-tip end. The tips come in different sizes, or gauges. The higher the gauge, the finer the point, which helps to get a blood sample less painfully. Even young children may be able to take their own blood samples, with adult supervision. To avoid spreading infections, your lancing device should not be used on anyone else.

Getting the Equipment
When you buy a glucose meter, there are a number of factors to consider. Most important, does your diabetes team have confidence in the accuracy of this meter? Other possible factors are the size of the meter and whether it's easy to take to school, to work or to the gym, the time required to perform a blood test, how much blood is required to get a reliable test result, how easy it is to operate the meter, what error messages you get if there is a problem with the test strip or the technique, how easy it is to calibrate the meter if necessary, whether the meter has memory capacity and whether it can be downloaded to a computer.

Whichever meter you prefer, consider how firmly the manufacturer stands behind its product. Does it provide a toll-free number for questions and technical support? Is the health care team familiar with this particular brand, should you have other questions?

Most glucose meters come as a kit that includes a finger-pricking or lancing device, a few check strips, control solution and a carrying case. It's much easier to get a blood sample with one of these devices than by using the lancet tip alone.

Ensuring Accuracy

To ensure that the glucose meter is working properly, it should be checked regularly with the check strips and control solution supplied with the system. At every visit, if possible—and at least once or twice a year—a blood glucose test should be done both in the lab and by your meter to check its accuracy. Results of the meter test should be within 10 to 15 percent of the lab test. For example, if the lab reading is 10 mmol/L (180 mg/dL), the meter result should be between 8.5 and 11.5 mmol/L (150–210 mg/dL).

Checking Urine

For Sugar

Because blood sugar checks are now the primary method of assessing diabetes control at home, urinary sugar is usually checked only as a back-up to checking blood sugar, or to screen other family members. A chemically treated strip is dipped briefly into a fresh urine sample. As with blood sugar checks, the strip will change color. After a defined period of time the strip is compared with a color chart on the box.

As discussed in Chapter One, when the blood sugar level exceeds the renal threshold (about 8.0–12.0 mmol/L, or 145–220 mg/dL), the kidneys filter out the excess sugar, which then appears in the urine. A urine check showing no sugar indicates that *when the urine was formed* the blood sugar level was below the renal threshold. If the urine shows sugar, the blood sugar was above the threshold when the urine was formed. These urine checks are at best an indirect measure of blood sugar, because the urine collected for the test may have been produced over a number of hours.

Checking urine for sugar is most useful as a screening tool for other members of the family, if they show signs of diabetes such as frequent and excessive urination. Because the blood sugar in people without diabetes generally does not exceed the renal threshold, sugar is not usually found in their urine. If sugar appears, further investigation is required.

For Ketones

Urinary ketones are tested in the same way as urinary sugar— by dipping a chemically treated strip in a fresh sample of urine, and comparing the color change to a chart. A purple color indicates ketones in the urine. Ketones are a sign of excessive breakdown of fat in the body. This can have a number of causes, including too little insulin or the stress of an illness. They may be detected in someone who doesn't have diabetes if the person is starving, or dieting to excess. In that case, though, the blood sugar level should be normal or low, rather than high.

Check urine ketones whenever:

- blood sugar level is over 13 mmol/L (230 mg/dL) for three readings in a row
- the child is feeling ill, has a fever or has vomited
- the child has symptoms of high blood sugar, i.e. increased thirst and urination
- the diabetes team asks you to check for ketones—perhaps when the insulin dose is being adjusted

Keep strips for ketone testing at home at all times. Ensure that the expiration date on the bottle has not passed, and that the bottle is kept closed.

Note that strips are available to check for ketones and sugar at the same time. Follow the instructions on the package carefully, and ask your health care team for help if the instructions are not clear.

Record-Keeping

The first step in spotting trends in glucose levels is to set up a logbook and complete it daily. Effective diabetes management is like putting the pieces of a puzzle together, and you can't complete the puzzle without all the pieces. Many pharmacies and pharmaceutical companies provide logbooks specially designed for diabetes management. Children can also make their own. A logbook should document:

- the amount and timing of each insulin injection
- the time and result of each blood sugar check
- the results of any urine tests for sugar and ketones
- any unusual circumstances related to the diabetes (i.e., a missed snack, a minor illness or strenuous activity and all insulin reactions—including the time of day and, if possible, the cause of the reaction)

Why all the effort? Accurate daily records will help parents, the child and the team decide when changes are needed in the insulin dose or meal plan. Be sure to record immediately the results of tests and the amounts of insulin given. These numbers are difficult to remember or to figure out after several days have gone by.

Children need help recording these measurements at first, but as they get older they should be able to maintain their own books. Check the book regularly to stay informed, and to make sure the child is recording daily measurements diligently. Record-keeping can be tedious, so don't be surprised if the

Sample logbook

Date	Insulin Type	Fasting	Before Noon Meal	Before Evening Meal	Bedtime	Other	Ketone Tests Results	Time	A.M. Meal	Noon Meal	P.M. Meal	Bedtime	Other	Notes
Mon. May 25	N / H	32 / 14	Ø / 14	22					6.8	12.4	7.6	5.7		morning math test
Tues. 26	N / H	32 / 14	Ø / 14	22					9.6	5.4	*3.2	11.7		* forgot afternoon snack
Wed. 27	N / H	32 / 14	Ø / 14	22					10.2	9.5	8.1	5.3		
Thurs. 28	N / H	32 / 14	Ø / 14	22					12.2	7.9	6.5	8.6		gym after lunch
Fri. 29	N / H	32 / 14	Ø / 14	22					14.0	9.2	12.4	7.3		
Sat. 30	N / H	32 / 14	Ø / 14	24			no ketones	7AM	18.6	11.1	8.7	9.4		
Sun. 31	N / H	32 / 14	Ø / 14						9.2	8.0	*5.9	12.9		reaction after basketball 4pm.

child needs help from time to time.

A number of glucose meters have memory to store the time and result of a given blood sugar check. As a result, it's tempting not to record results right away because "it's all in the meter." This can be a problem. Although the meter's memory capabilities may mean that you don't have to download results into the logbook as often, the meter doesn't replace the logbook. Without a well-kept record, it is almost impossible to recognize patterns of blood sugar levels and to make appropriate adjustments in a timely way.

Hemoglobin A1c (HbA1c) Testing— The Three-month Test

The hemoglobin A_{1c} test is a measure of average blood sugar level over the previous three months. This test is also known as *glycosylated* or *glycated hemoglobin* or *glycohemoglobin*. Hemoglobin is the part of the red blood cell that carries oxygen from the lungs to the rest of the body. Scientists have discovered that in all people, whether they have diabetes or not, some sugar sticks to the hemoglobin and stays there for the lifespan of the red blood cell—about three to four months. The amount of sugar that sticks to the hemoglobin reflects the average blood sugar level during that period, and can be measured in a laboratory using the HbA_{1c} test. When the average blood sugar level has been high, the test result will be high. Thus, the HbA_{1c} indicates the level of control over the previous few months.

HbA_{1c} can be measured at any time, and often enough blood can be collected for this test from a finger prick, although sometimes the blood sample has to be taken from a vein. There are different methods for measuring HbA_{1c}. Some give immediate results, others take a day or more. HbA_{1c} in people without diabetes is about 4 to 6 percent (0.04–0.06); check the non-diabetic range for your laboratory. Even with intensive treatment, few children and teens with diabetes can achieve this level without risking frequent low blood sugar reactions. Instead, strive to achieve the best HbA_{1c} levels possible. In the absence of many low blood sugar reactions, levels from 6 to 7 percent are considered excellent, while those between 7 and 8 percent are very good. Levels between 8 and 10 percent suggest a need for extra effort to improve control, and levels over 10 percent indicate a need for concerted effort by child, family and team to avoid trouble.

Children should have their HbA$_{1c}$ measured every three months and the results should be recorded to chart overall progress. Be sure to note when a different lab than the usual one processes the test—methods, and therefore results, can differ from lab to lab, giving an inaccurate picture of progress.

What HbAlc levels mean in terms of average blood sugar concentrations

HbAlc	mmol/L	mg/dL
5%	5.0	90
6%	6.5–7.0	115–125
7%	8.0–9.0	145–160
8%	9.5–11.0	170–200
9%	11.0–13.0	200–240
10%	12.5–15.0	230–270
11%	14.0–17.0	250–300
12%	15.5–19.0	280–350

Adjusting Insulin Doses

As children grow and their appetites and activity levels change, their need for insulin also changes. You shouldn't have to wait for a regular appointment with someone on the diabetes team to respond to these changes. Who better to monitor the changing patterns in the child's blood glucose level and overall health than the family? Studies show that parents and children who actively participate in the diabetes management process are the most successful in adapting to the disease.

Remember that the need for more insulin or more injections does *not* mean a child's diabetes is getting worse. Similarly, a decrease in insulin doesn't mean the diabetes is going away. Adjusting insulin to the body's current demands is simply a way of maintaining good balance and achieving better control. For example, a heavier child may need more insulin than a smaller child, and a child who is always on the go may need less insulin than a child who is not as active. An adolescent may require more insulin during exam week, to compensate for increased stress. A teenager will likely require more insulin during puberty than after the growth spurt.

To make independent insulin adjustments, parents and teens must:

- be confident that blood glucose checks are accurate and meal plans are being followed (i.e. no secret snacking)
- be confident of the child's blood glucose target range
- understand the actions of the insulin being used
- understand what each blood sugar check means
- know when to contact the health care team

When to Make Adjustments

People with diabetes know when change is in order by the way they feel, and by the results of their blood sugar or urine ketone checks. Provided that they are sticking to the meal plan closely, continuous high blood sugar readings usually mean that more insulin is required; repeated low readings usually mean that less insulin is required. Generally speaking, you can assume that the insulin dose is right and no change is necessary when:

- the child feels well and is free of symptoms of high or low blood sugar
- the urine is free of ketones
- 70–80 percent of the blood sugar checks are within the target range

With any insulin regimen, be it two, three or four injections a day, it is important to know which insulin is acting when, and therefore which insulin dose needs to be adjusted when sugar levels are either too high or too low.

Jane is a 10-year-old who has had diabetes for five years. She receives NPH and Regular insulin before breakfast, Regular at supper and NPH at bedtime. Jane's family has learned that each of the four daily blood checks is dependent on the action of one of the four insulin doses:
- the breakfast reading tells them how well the bedtime NPH from the night before is working
- the lunch reading indicates the effectiveness of the breakfast Regular insulin
- the supper reading reflects the action of the breakfast NPH
- the bedtime reading tells them if the supper Regular insulin is working

These guidelines may seem a little simplistic, but they're a good starting point for Jane and her family when her blood checks are off target. When Jane woke up with high readings three mornings in a row, her parents knew she needed more NPH (intermediate-acting) insulin at night. When she had a couple of nights when she was low before her bedtime snack, her parents decreased her Regular (fast-acting) dose at suppertime.

Pattern Management
Most people aim to keep blood sugar levels in the target range 70–80 percent of the time. Some variability is to be expected. The insulin dose should be changed only when a pattern or trend of off-target blood sugar appears: when the blood sugar is high at the same time of day for three days in a row, or low at the same time of day more than twice a week or two days in a row. As long as the child is feeling well and is free of ketones, wait until the checks have been outside the target range three times for highs and twice for lows, before adjusting the insulin dose.

You should also check for ketones if the blood glucose is above 13 mmol/L (230 mg/dL) for three consecutive readings. Ketones in the urine along with blood sugar above this level may indicate the need for more immediate adjustment. Consult the diabetes doctor or nurse immediately if this occurs. Here are some guidelines for insulin dose adjustment, for children or teens on a mixture of intermediate (NPH/Lente) and fast-acting or superfast-acting (Regular or Lispro) pre-breakfast insulin, fast-acting or superfast-acting pre-supper insulin and intermediate-acting insulin at bedtime. Apply them only on the advice of a doctor.

If high	before breakfast	*increase*	bedtime intermediate
(at any one	before lunch		morning fast/superfast
of these times	before supper		morning intermediate
3 days in	before bedtime		supper fast/superfast
a row)	snack		

If low	before breakfast	*decrease*	bedtime intermediate
(at any one	before lunch		morning fast/superfast
of these times	before supper		morning intermediate
more than	before bedtime		supper fast/superfast
twice a week	snack		
or 2 days in			
a row)			

- Change the insulin dosage by only 10 percent as often as every other day until one of the checks falls within the target range.
- If the total insulin dose has been increased by 10 units and no blood sugar level is within the target range, contact the doctor or diabetes nurse before making further adjustments.

What does a 10 percent dose adjustment mean?

If the child is on:	adjust by:
less than 20 units of insulin/day	1 unit at a time
20–30 units/day	2 units at a time
30–40 units/day	3 units at a time
over 40 units/day	4 units at a time

Variable Insulin Dose Schedule—"The Sliding Scale"

Many children and teens with diabetes receive a fixed amount of intermediate-acting insulin, but vary the amount of fast- (or superfast-) acting insulin depending on the blood sugar reading at the time of the injection—more insulin for higher and less insulin for lower readings. This allows gentle corrections to prevent long periods of highs or lows. In general, a basic amount of fast-acting insulin is prescribed for blood sugar levels that fall in the target range, a unit or two are removed for readings below target, and one to four units are added as levels increase above target.

In addition to using the scale to correct highs or lows, you can learn to make further adjustments to compensate for rigorous activities, or a change in meal plan over the next three to four hours.

Note that even when a variable dose schedule is used, you still need to watch for patterns and respond to them, so that you can make appropriate adjustments.

Consider Tom's variable scale (see box below). His target range is 4.0–10.0. If Tom's pre-supper blood sugar result is 13.1 and Tom is on Lispro insulin, the scale indicates that the dose Tom should take this evening is 7+1 = 8 units Lispro. However, if Tom is going to play tennis right after supper he may decide

Sample of variable insulin dose scale

Blood Sugar	breakfast		Insulin supper	bed
	L	**N**	**L**	**N**
<3.0	−2		−2	
3.1–3.9	−1		−1	
4.0–10.0	5	17	7	10
10.1–14.0	+1		+1	
14.1–17.0	+2		+2	
>17.0	+3		+3	
(**L** = Lispro, **N** = NPH)				

(on the basis of experience and discussion with his health care team) to reduce his Lispro by two units, so his dose will be 7+1–2 = 6 units.

"Intensive" Diabetes Management

Intensive diabetes management is intended to maintain blood sugar levels as close to non-diabetic levels as possible. The target range is tightened to 4–7 mmol/L (70–125 mg/dL) before meals. For what purpose? When blood sugar is maintained at lower levels over the years, the risk of developing the long-term complications of diabetes, such as eye or kidney disease, is reduced. This becomes increasingly important once puberty has begun.

Traditional or conventional diabetes management consists of taking insulin two or three times a day, monitoring blood sugar two to four times a day, following a meal plan that involves eating the same amount of food at around the same time each day and compensating for extra activity with extra food or sometimes less insulin.

Intensive diabetes management is a more proactive approach. And while it requires careful attention to meals and exercise planning, intensive management allows a more flexible schedule. It's like flying a jumbo jet compared to a one-engine plane—it may be more complex but there is also more potential. People can vary their activities more, and don't have to eat meals at the same time every day because they are taking insulin before every meal. Through either four or five daily injections, or an insulin infusion pump, intensive therapy aims to provide a steady stream of insulin throughout the day—more the way a pancreas does—with extra insulin at mealtime.

Here's how it works. Fast-acting or superfast-acting insulin is usually taken three times a day—before breakfast, lunch and dinner. Intermediate-acting insulin is taken at bedtime. The dose of the fast-acting insulin is based on the current blood sugar level. Thus, when blood sugar goes higher than 7 mmol/L (125 mg/dL) before a given meal, there is an opportunity to give some extra fast-acting or superfast-acting insulin right then, to bring the blood sugar back into the target range. Likewise, if the blood sugar level is under 4 mmol/L (70 mg/dL) just prior to a meal, or if a lot of exercise is planned in the next few hours, the insulin dose can be reduced immediately.

Intensive diabetes management was central to the ground-breaking Diabetes Control and Complications Trial (DCCT)—a multicenter U.S.-government-funded study that looked at the effects of tight blood sugar control on the risk of diabetes complications. In this study, more than 1,400 volunteers were divided into two groups. One group managed their diabetes with intensive therapy, while the other group continued with traditional therapy. At the end of the nine-year period, the two groups were compared. The intensive therapy group showed an average HbA_{1c} reading of 7.2 percent, significantly lower than the traditional treatment group's average of 8.9 percent. The intensive therapy group had fewer signs of complications from diabetes: diabetic eye disease (retinopathy) had started in only one-quarter as many people as in the control group; kidney disease (nephropathy) occurred in only half as many; nerve disease (neuropathy) in only one-third as many. And of those under intensive management who showed early signs of these three complications before the study began, far fewer showed progression of the complications.

Intensive diabetes management isn't for everybody, however. The DCCT involved only teens and adults. The benefit of intensive treatment for younger children has not yet been proved. Attempting to keep blood sugar levels closer to normal increases the risk of low blood sugar or insulin reactions. The volunteers in the DCCT who used intensive management reported hypoglycemic reactions three times as often as those using conventional therapy. For those unable to recognize and treat their own hypoglycemia, such as the very young, intensive treatment could be dangerous.

Families who choose this approach must prepare themselves for the extra work, and make sure they have the support of their diabetes team. If a young person is already achieving fairly tight control with standard therapy (i.e. HbA_{1c} less than about 7.5 percent), there may be little overall benefit from switching. Similarly, those with high hemoglobin A_{1c} results— 10 percent or more—may want to bone up on standard therapy before making the leap to intensive therapy. All the same, there is no doubt that intensive therapy is fast becoming the standard of care for teens and adults with Type 1 diabetes.

Adjusting Insulin and Food for Planned Activity

Most children welcome routines, but once in a while schedules change, and without adequate planning the blood sugar balance may be upset. A weekly swimming lesson on Sunday morning, for example, will create different insulin demands than a weekly piano lesson on Monday afternoon. Parents, and in time children, can learn to assess the impact of these regular events, and when an opportunity for a new activity comes along, everyone will be better able to cope with the change.

Because exercise both lowers blood glucose and increases the speed of insulin absorption, it's a good idea to match it, whenever possible, with extra food. After a while, you'll become more familiar with how the child responds to activity and you'll have a better idea of how much food, if any, to offer. Some (usually older) children learn to decrease insulin on days of extra activity rather than taking extra food.

- In general, provide extra food for extra exercise. Children need about 10 to 15 grams of carbohydrate (such as a four-ounce, or 125 mL, juice box, or half a sandwich) for every 30 minutes of activity outside the usual. If possible, monitor blood glucose levels before and after the activity—these levels will provide important information for future activities. For example, if the sugar level is very high after an activity, then less (or no) extra food may be needed. If the sugar level is low, even more snacks will be required.

- Always make sure children have enough food with them (such as glucose tablets, fruit roll-ups, juice boxes or granola bars), especially if the activity goes on a long time or is off the beaten track.

- If the child starts to experience a low blood sugar reaction, stop the activity immediately and treat the reaction. Don't resume the activity until the symptoms have resolved and the child has eaten some extra food.

Preventing Delayed Low Blood Sugar
- Monitor blood glucose levels long after exercise. Lows can occur up to 12 hours later.

- Children doing activities after supper should have a bigger evening snack. Doing a midnight or middle-of-the-night (two to four a.m.) check will help detect late-night lows.

Twelve-year-old Michele has always taken her ballet lesson on Saturday afternoon. To get ready for an exam, she's planning to add an extra hour to the lesson. In preparation for the change in her schedule, Michele's parents consider her current routine. Michele always has an afternoon snack of a fruit and starch. The extended class means that she'll be dancing at the time when her morning intermediate-acting (NPH) insulin is reaching its peak. Michele will be home for her usual six p.m. supper. Without the extra class, her blood glucose level is usually between 8 and 12 mmol/L (145–220 mg/dL) at suppertime. However, her blood glucose level often drops in the night after vigorous exercise late in the day. Michele's parents work out the following plan:

- Eat an extra fruit and starch choice prior to her second hour of dance.
- Take blood glucose monitoring equipment to the lesson, as well as a small juice box and granola bar, in case her blood glucose starts to drop during the lesson.
- Check the blood glucose level at the end of the class to evaluate the effectiveness of the plan.
- Eat an additional starch choice at bedtime to offset the delayed effects of the exercise.

Q&A

My 15-year-old daughter's pre-dinner blood sugar checks are either high or missing most of the time. I suspect that she's snacking on the way home from school and that's why her blood sugar is a little high. Any ideas about how to approach this?

You're wise not to demand explanations for why every test result is the way it is—or to accuse your daughter of cheating. This is a sure way to get no blood sugar readings, or "made up" results. On the other hand, it is risky to increase the insulin dose if you're not confident that the readings are accurate. It could be that the checks are done just a short while after your daughter has been snacking. Some parents deal with this situation by saying to their teen, "It seems your blood sugar checks are high before supper. Let's put our heads together to figure out what kinds of adjustments might be necessary." This gives you an opportunity to explore some of the factors that may be contributing to the high level, such as being hungry and eating more right after school or on the way home. Then the right kind of adjustments can be made.

Should I let my son continue to play in day-long soccer tournaments? What about the walk-a-thon next month?
If your son played in day-long soccer tournaments before he was diagnosed with diabetes, then by all means continue. One of the most important steps in helping children cope with diabetes is minimizing change in their lifestyle. Even if all-day soccer tournaments are new to his list of activities, there's still no need to ban them. If you cut out soccer tournaments, something your son presumably enjoys, you'll increase any resentment he may have toward the disease, and perhaps toward you. You can prepare him for a day-long tournament, or next month's walk-a-thon, by providing lots of snacks and monitoring his blood sugar in as subtle a way as possible. To start, at least, you should also give a little less insulin on these days. Once you see the effect of the extra activity on his glucose levels, you can decide whether less insulin, more food or a combination of both is the best way to go. Consult your diabetes team for more advice.

Is it all right to scuba dive?
For a long time scuba diving was considered too dangerous for people with diabetes, because of the risk of becoming hypoglycemic under water and not being able to respond by taking sugar, causing a mild insulin reaction to escalate into a severe one. However, researchers are finding that hard and fast restrictions don't work, and further studies are being done. At present, divers with diabetes are advised to consult a doctor experienced in dive medicine, to learn everything they can about taking the necessary safety precautions. Make sure that you recognize the risks involved, and that your dive buddy knows the risks too. For the latest information on the subject, call the Divers Alert Network (DAN) at Duke University Medical Center, at 919-684-2948, ext. 222. Or check their webpage at http://jshaldane.mc.duke.edu/Projects/DADindex.htm.

Every time my blood sugar is high, my mom sends me outside to run around the block. Meanwhile my sister sits in front of the TV. It doesn't seem fair.
Your mom is concerned about the effects of your high blood sugar, and it sounds as if she's using exercise as a way to help you bring it down. However, perhaps you and your mom could sit down and figure out other ways to bring down your blood sugar. For instance, if this is happening at the same time every day, maybe you need to increase the insulin dose that would affect this sugar reading.

My teenage daughter thinks she's too heavy. She's been exercising four to six hours a day trying to lose weight. Is this healthy for her?
No. Most people do not lose weight when they increase their activity level—they seem to take in an increased amount of

food to offset the fuel burned by the exercise. Excessive amounts of exercise in a teenage girl wanting to lose weight may be one of the first signs that she is unduly worried about her body image and possibly developing an eating disorder. Discuss your concern with your family doctor and members of your diabetes team.

Our family is very athletic, and I expect our six-year-old son has a lot of potential too. How can we encourage him to explore athletics without being intimidated by his diabetes? Introduce your son to sports slowly, and increase his exposure as he shows more interest. Many professional and skilled amateur athletes have diabetes. Your local support group should be able to provide a list. Encourage your son to write to athletes with diabetes and to use them as role models. Many athletes find the time to write a note back, which can be all the encouragement a child needs.

SIX

Handling Highs and Lows

Jacob knew he should stop and take a break from the squash game, but he was having too much fun. And besides, he was winning for a change. "Are you sure you don't want to stop and have some juice?" his brother Paul asked. "You've been working pretty hard." "You're just trying to avoid losing," Jacob kidded. A few minutes passed and Paul insisted they stop for a juice break. "Look, I know when I need a break," said Jacob sharply, no longer kidding. "Let's just keep playing." Suddenly he was feeling a little light-headed and weak in the knees. Paul noticed that Jacob was getting paler and paler and ran to get some orange juice from his sports bag. Within a few minutes Jacob's color began to return to normal.

Jacob has a low blood sugar reaction at least once or twice a week. Most of the time he recognizes them and treats them without incident. But sometimes, when he gets caught up in friendly competition, he pushes himself beyond safe limits. Luckily, his brother knew the signs—first angry and defensive, then clammy and faint. If he hadn't got treatment at that point,

Jacob might have become confused, drowsy and unable to take anything by mouth.

It's been said that managing diabetes is a little like performing a juggling act while sitting on a horse charging forward. Sometimes the ball drops. No matter how hard you try, it's impossible to keep the blood sugar in target range all of the time. Sometimes it will be high, other times low. Often there is no explanation for the results. This chapter covers the extremes:

- *hypoglycemia*, or low blood sugar, often referred to as an insulin reaction or insulin shock
- *diabetic ketoacidosis (DKA)*, the result of a severe shortage of insulin
- *sick days*, leading to either hypoglycemia or DKA when not handled properly

Hypoglycemia (Low Blood Sugar or Insulin Reaction)

A blood sugar level lower than about 3.3 mmol/L (60 mg/dL) is defined as hypoglycemia. The feelings associated with hypoglycemia are called an "insulin reaction."

The earliest symptoms of low blood sugar may resemble the feelings many people experience when they've gone without food for a long time: they may feel hungry, tired and irritable, and may even have a headache. These early warning signs tell us that the body needs sugar quickly. As the blood sugar continues to drop, other signs and symptoms may develop—shakiness, pale skin, cold sweat, dilated pupils and pounding heart. These result from the body's attempt to boost the blood sugar from within. Certain hormones, including glucagon, adrenaline, cortisol and others, urge our liver and muscles to convert stored sugar into glucose, which enters the bloodstream.

In someone without diabetes, the body turns off the insulin supply whenever blood sugar is at a normal level, or below normal. But in people with diabetes, the injected insulin continues to work; as fast as the glucose enters the bloodstream, the insulin pushes it into the cells, so the level of sugar in the blood remains low until the person takes sugar by mouth.

Most people with Type 1 diabetes experience low blood sugar reactions from time to time. Indeed, mild reactions that are easily recognized and treated, without too much interruption in activities, should be expected. They can be seen as the price paid for good blood glucose control. Note that some people experience symptoms of hypoglycemia even when their blood sugar level is higher than 3.3 mmol/L.

Common Signs and Symptoms of a Mild Insulin Reaction

- shakiness—"butterflies," feeling nervous for no reason
- cold, clammy sweatiness, unlike sweat from playing hard
- dilated pupils, "funny-looking" eyes
- mood change—irritable, grouchy, impatient; temper tantrums in younger children
- xhunger, and sometimes nausea due to the hunger
- lack of energy—tired, weak, floppy
- lack of concentration
- blurred vision
- pounding heart
- change in skin color—pale, most noticeably in the face and around the mouth
- poor sleep patterns—restlessness, crying out, sleepwalking or nightmares

Usually insulin reactions happen suddenly, over a period of minutes rather than hours. While they may occur at any time of the day or night, they happen most often when insulin is working at its peak.

Although low blood sugar symptoms vary from child to child, each child tends to develop his or her own set of symptoms. After one or two episodes, parents and children learn to recognize an insulin reaction quickly. It is helpful for parents and older children to explain the child's specific symptoms to teachers, coaches, school bus drivers and other caregivers. Even young children can be taught to alert an adult to these symptoms, by using a specific phrase such as "I feel funny" or "I need sugar."

Hypoglycemia may be most difficult to detect in infants or toddlers, who are unable to describe their feelings. A sudden change in behavior, with irritability, crying, pale face and "floppiness," may be the tip-off that hypoglycemia is setting in.

Treatment of Mild Insulin Reaction
Insulin reactions, even mild ones, must be treated right away. Always have a source of fast-acting sugar available, such as juice, dextrose tablets or even table sugar. In the event of an insulin reaction, follow these steps:
- If possible, check the blood sugar level to confirm hypoglycemia. A blood glucose level lower than 6 mmol/L (110 mg/dL), *accompanied by* symptoms of low blood sugar, should be treated. (If you are unable to check the blood sugar before treating the reaction, check it as soon as possible afterward. Note the response to treatment.)
- Give a source of quick-acting sugar; about 10–15 grams of carbohydrate is all it takes to treat an insulin reaction. Examples include: four ounces (125 mL) of unsweetened

juice or regular soft drink, or two to three dextrose tablets, or eight ounces (250 mL) of milk, or 2 teaspoons (10 mL) of sugar. Various forms of prepackaged glucose gel may also be available from your pharmacy or diabetes supply shop. Read the label ahead of time to determine the amount you should give to treat a low blood sugar reaction. We generally recommend an amount that will supply 10–15 grams of carbohydrate. If a mild reaction occurs just before a meal or snack, start the meal or snack, beginning with some simple carbohydrate.

- Wait for the sugar to take effect. This is the hardest part. People who experience hypoglycemia feel extremely hungry and scared. They are often tempted to continue to eat and drink until the symptoms go away. This may result in a high blood sugar level later in the day. If symptoms persist, recheck the blood sugar in 10 to 15 minutes. If it is still low, the child should have an extra 10–15 grams of carbohydrate. If vigorous exercise is anticipated prior to the next meal or snack, or if the reaction occurs during the night, the simple carbohydrate should be followed with a complex carbohydrate (one from the starch category).
- Attempt to determine the cause, if any, of the insulin reaction. If there is no apparent reason, consider reducing the appropriate insulin by 10 to 20 percent the next day. As much as we seek the reasons for a hypoglycemic reaction, sometimes there is no obvious cause.
- Note the blood sugar levels, time, response and possible cause of the reaction in your record book.

Note: if in doubt, treat. When you can't check the blood sugar level to confirm an insulin reaction, a sugar source should be given to be safe.

Why Do Insulin Reactions Occur?

Understanding the reasons for hypoglycemia is key to preventing it. Causes are usually related to the three major factors affecting blood sugar balance: insulin, food and activity.

Too Much Insulin

Children can get too much insulin if the wrong amount is given; if the parents or the child inadvertently give a dose at the wrong time, such as giving the pre-breakfast dose at suppertime; or if the dose isn't reduced when blood sugar readings are consistently less than the target level.

Not Enough Food

This can happen easily enough—for example, when children get caught up in their activities and forget to eat, when toddlers sleep through snack time or when teens sleep through breakfast or skip a meal.

Too Much Unplanned Activity

This is the most frequent cause of hypoglycemia, because children aren't accustomed to planning ahead before they jump into an active game like tag or football. That's why the blood glucose target range is wider in younger children than in adults; it allows for such spontaneity. Children should be able to enjoy any sport or activity with planning.

Severe Hypoglycemic Reaction

Occasionally a severe hypoglycemic reaction—insulin shock—occurs when early symptoms of low blood sugar go undetected and untreated. Know what to look for and what to do in case a severe low blood sugar reaction develops.

Signs and Symptoms of a Severe Insulin Reaction
- "drunken-like behavior"—slurred speech, staggering, confusion, combativeness
- low energy—extremely tired, difficult to wake up
- loss of consciousness
- convulsions or seizures
- temporary paralysis down one side of the body

Treatment of a Severe Insulin Reaction

This is an emergency situation. Anyone showing signs of severe insulin reaction needs immediate help. The blood sugar is dangerously low, therefore the child needs sugar. However, someone who is very drowsy, unconscious or having a convulsion or seizure must not be given juice or any other liquid by mouth, because of the risk of choking. Rather, the child should be turned onto his or her side to prevent choking, and glucagon should be injected. If a glucagon emergency kit is not available, an ambulance should be called and the child transported to the closest hospital emergency department, where either a glucose-containing solution will be injected intravenously, or glucagon will be given. While you wait for the ambulance, honey, corn syrup or a glucose gel may be rubbed on the lips, gums or lining of the child's mouth. Some of the glucose in these products may be absorbed without the child having to swallow.

About Glucagon

Glucagon is a hormone that stimulates the liver to release sugar into the bloodstream. It must be injected; if it's taken by mouth, it's digested and doesn't reach the bloodstream. When glucagon acts on the liver, the blood sugar level rises and the symptoms usually disappear within about 15 minutes. Families of all children with Type 1 diabetes should have usable (not expired) glucagon on hand, and know where it's kept and how to use it. A glucagon emergency kit consists of a small vial containing dry glucagon powder and a pre-filled glass syringe containing sterile diluting solution. The contents of the syringe and vial should be mixed only when they are about to be used. Keep the kit in an agreed-upon place so everyone can find it easily.

An injection of glucagon can never be harmful. It is impossible to overdose on glucagon. Parents who think their child may need glucagon should play it safe and give the injection.

Preparing and Giving Glucagon

- Remove the flip-off seal from the vial (bottle) of glucagon.
- Remove the needle protector from the syringe and inject the entire contents of the syringe into the vial of glucagon.
- Remove the syringe. Shake vial gently until glucagon dissolves and the solution becomes clear.
- Using the same syringe, withdraw all of the solution from the vial.
- For children six years of age and older, inject all of the solution, just as you would inject insulin. Children under six may require only half the mixed dose, as recommended by the doctor or diabetes nurse.

After the glucagon has been injected, check the blood glucose and observe the child carefully. He or she should wake up in 5 to 20 minutes. If not, the child should be taken to the closest hospital emergency department. Once the child is fully awake, offer some juice or a sugar-containing soft drink. Recheck the blood sugar if possible and notify the doctor. It is likely that the insulin dose should be reduced significantly.

Either the severe hypoglycemic reaction or the use of

glucagon can trigger nausea or vomiting, especially in children. They may be unable to eat or drink afterward. If this occurs:

- Recheck blood sugar levels immediately.
- If you are able to reach the doctor, he or she can advise you on whether to proceed to the hospital.
- If you cannot reach the doctor and the child does not stop vomiting, go to the nearest hospital, even if the blood glucose levels are starting to rise.

Remember, a glucagon kit doesn't do any good if no one knows where it's kept or how to use it.

Reducing the Risk of Hypoglycemia
Low blood sugar reactions are not always preventable, but there are things you can do to keep them to a minimum.

- *Eat meals and snacks on time.* A delay of half an hour or more can result in hypoglycemia.
- *Make sure that the proper insulin dose is prepared and given.* Children require close supervision with this task.
- *Plan for extra activity with extra food or an insulin reduction.* Set up a good communication system with teachers, coaches and other leaders so you'll know when extra activity is planned.
- *Negotiate realistic blood sugar targets with your health care team.* For example, it may be inappropriate and even dangerous to aim for "normal" blood sugar levels in very young children.
- *Remember to lower the insulin dose* if the sugar level is low at the same time of day two days in a row, or twice in a week.
- *Always have some form of quick-acting sugar close by—* and make sure everyone knows where it is.

- Make sure that teens are aware that *drinking alcohol can cause hypoglycemia.*
- *Keep a glucagon emergency kit at home.* Review its use regularly. Take it with you on vacation. Replace it when it reaches its expiry date, and practice preparing it before you throw it out.
- Encourage your child to *wear medical-alert identification,* and to carry a wallet card if older.

False Low Blood Sugar Reactions
Sometimes children feel anxious, nervous or tired and think it's due to low blood sugar when it isn't. There are many reasons for this. A quick blood sugar check is the best way to find out whether or not the blood sugar is low. Sometimes low blood sugar symptoms occur when the blood sugar drops quickly from a high to a normal level. Feeling nervous or upset for other reasons, such as exams, can also be confused with hypoglycemia. And occasionally the symptoms of high blood sugar are mistaken for a low sugar reaction. Once the blood glucose has been checked and it is clear that the result is not low, reassure the child that he or she can resume the activity. However, if in doubt, treat the symptoms.

High Blood Sugar (Hyperglycemia)
Parents of children with diabetes quickly discover that, no matter how much they know about the disease, and no matter how hard they try to get excellent blood sugar results, the levels will be high from time to time. This is to be expected. Sometimes the reasons are obvious—a test done too soon after the last meal or snack; a lazy rainy day; an extra treat at a birthday party; or some insulin leakage from an injection site. Often, however, there's no obvious reason for the high level, which

will seem unfair to those who invest a lot of time and effort in controlling blood sugar. But it's no one's fault. It's just the result of an imperfect means of replacing insulin. Injecting insulin even three or four times a day does not restore the automatic blood sugar regulation that people without diabetes take for granted. There will never be a perfect match between the blood sugar and the injected insulin. There will be occasional highs regardless of how careful you are.

Blood sugar results on their own do not tell the whole story. Parents should also want to know if their child:

- is experiencing any symptoms of hyperglycemia, such as thirst, increased urination or fatigue
- is showing signs of being sick, such as a cough or fever
- has ketones in the urine

An isolated high blood sugar level—even one in the high teens or twenties (300–400 mg/dL)—is no cause for concern as long as the child feels well and there are no ketones in the urine. If high blood sugar levels persist, even in the absence of symptoms or ketones, an insulin adjustment may be required. (See Chapter Five.)

A high blood sugar level combined with either ketones in the urine or the signs and symptoms of high blood sugar indicates a need for immediate action. Additional fast-acting insulin (Regular or Lispro) should be injected. The diabetes team will help you decide how much insulin to give. Failure to take action when the blood sugar level is high and ketones are present can lead to diabetic ketoacidosis, a life-threatening condition.

High Blood Sugar Symptoms
- urinating more than usual (polyuria)
- getting up in the night to urinate (nocturia)

- bedwetting (enuresis)
- thirst (polydipsia)
- poor energy level, tired and irritable (and doesn't get better with food)
- blurred vision
- weight loss

Diabetic Ketoacidosis (DKA)

DKA develops when there is a serious lack of insulin in the body. This may occur at the time of diagnosis (some 10 to 25 percent of children with newly diagnosed diabetes have arrived in the emergency room with DKA) or if one of two situations arises:

- failure to take any or enough insulin
- failure to take sufficient extra insulin to cover the high sugar and ketone production caused by infection or other illness

With insufficient insulin available, blood sugar levels rise and excess sugar spills into the urine. Then the body starts breaking down fat as an alternative supply of energy. The ketones produced by fat breakdown are acidic, causing ketoacidosis. As the condition worsens, and more and more water is lost in the urine and through vomiting, the child becomes increasingly dehydrated. DKA can be avoided by careful attention to all aspects of the diabetes treatment plan.

DKA usually develops over hours or days. Watch for:
- high blood sugar levels and ketones in the urine
- excessive thirst
- urinating much more often and in larger amounts
- sudden loss of weight
- complaints of stomach pains or nausea
- vomiting

- leg cramps
- a flushed appearance
- headache
- signs of dehydration: dry mouth and tongue, sore throat, dark circles under the eyes
- deep, heavy breathing, fruity-smelling breath
- drowsiness leading in time to unconsciousness

If a child exhibits any of these signs, the blood sugar level should be checked along with the presence of urinary ketones. Notify the doctor right away. DKA must be treated in a hospital.

Preventing DKA

Since one of the main reasons for developing DKA is failure to get enough insulin, clearly parents need to ensure that children and teens are getting the right amount of insulin at the right time. This responsibility is too much for a young child to assume alone. The other high-risk time for developing DKA is when the body is under stress due to fever—infection or flu, for example. These common conditions can become life-threatening if they are not adequately managed by the family with the support of their health care team. Become very familiar with the sick-day guidelines that follow, and remember—if you're taking a vacation, don't leave home without them.

Sick Days

Children with diabetes do not experience more illnesses than their non-diabetic friends, and should not miss more school days just because of their diabetes. An otherwise healthy person with *well-controlled* diabetes has normal resistance to infection. When diabetes is adequately controlled, injuries are not slow to heal. However, while illness may not be more likely, or more difficult to treat in a person with diabetes, *any* illness may upset the blood sugar balance.

When children with diabetes get sick, their blood sugar often goes high and ketones may show in the urine. Illness is a stress to the body, and stress creates a demand for more insulin. People without diabetes automatically make more insulin at such times. Children with diabetes do not. So on a sick day the usual amount of insulin may not be enough, and monitoring may show high blood sugar, with or without ketones. At such times you may need to increase the insulin dose, even though the appetite may be poor, to prevent DKA.

Although all illnesses in people with diabetes must be taken seriously, not all illnesses make the blood sugar go up. In fact, illnesses like diarrhea may be accompanied by low blood sugar levels. Careful monitoring of blood glucose levels and urinary ketones will help determine the effect of each illness and the appropriate response.

What to Do When a Child with Diabetes Is Ill

- Check the *blood sugar and urinary ketone levels* when the illness first appears (a mild case of the sniffles doesn't warrant checking, but a more severe cold or cough does) and continue to check every four hours around the clock.
- *Continue administering insulin.* Even though the child may not be eating well, the physical stress of the illness will probably raise the blood sugar level and cause ketones to form. Thus more insulin may be needed, rather than less. If the sugar levels go lower, less (but never no) insulin may be required. Remember that insulin is *always* required to prevent the breakdown of body fat into ketones.
- If the child doesn't want to eat, *give clear fluids containing sugar.* Offer small amounts of fruit juice, frozen ice treats, sugar-containing fruit-flavored gelatin or soft drinks frequently. Use the Two-Thirds Fluid Diet (see box).

• Teens with diabetes who are doing their own monitoring and insulin administration should be *helped or supervised* carefully throughout the illness.

• Be sure to *treat the underlying illness* that is upsetting diabetes control. Give the medications prescribed. Acetaminophen in the usual doses for fever or pain is safe unless the doctor says otherwise.

The Two-Thirds Fluid Diet

When a child with diabetes is sick and nauseated or doesn't want to eat the usual diet, a diet that is two-thirds fluid is recommended. This means that only two-thirds of the usual amount of carbohydrates are given on a sick day, and the diet is offered in the form of clear fluids, such as frozen ice treats, juice, sugar-containing fruit-flavored gelatin and soft drinks. With this diet children get enough carbohydrate, or sugar, to balance the insulin and produce energy.

The following table will help you decide how much sugar-containing fluid to offer on a sick day. Don't offer all the fluids for one meal at the same time. The fluids designated for breakfast can be consumed throughout the morning until lunch. Lunch-time fluids should be taken through the afternoon, and suppertime fluids through the evening.

No. of calories usually taken	No. of fruit choices to be given for each meal (breakfast, lunch, supper) on sick days
1000–1200	3–4
1200–1500	4–5
1500–2000	5–6
2000–2400	6.5–7.5
2400–3000	8.5–10.5
3000–3600	10.5–12

For example, someone on an 1800-calorie diet should have six fruit choices as clear fluids through the morning, and again in the afternoon and again in the evening. A fruit choice in fluid form may be any one of the following:

• 2 1/2 oz./80 mL apple juice
• 3 oz./100 mL unsweetened orange juice
• 2 1/2 oz./ 80 mL regular fruit-flavored gelatin
• 3 oz./100 mL (one-third can) regular ginger ale (not sugarless or diet)
• half an ice pop

• *Telephone the diabetes doctor or nurse immediately* if illness is accompanied by:
  – vomiting
  – eating or drinking poorly
  – urinary ketones
  – blood sugar above 17 mmol/L (300 mg/dL)

Note: if the child vomits twice or more within 12 hours, call the diabetes team or take the child to the hospital immediately.

Insulin Management during Illness

When children are sick they still need insulin at their usual times. In fact, they may require extra injections of fast-acting or superfast-acting insulin as often as every four hours, if they show high blood sugar or urine ketones. To decide how much insulin to give, check the blood sugar and urine ketones every four hours and consult this chart each time. The following illness scenarios offer courses of action depending on results of the blood glucose and urinary ketone tests.

Blood glucose	*Urine ketones*	*Action*
• 6.0–17.0 mmol/L (110–300 mg/dL)	negative or small	Give the usual insulin at the usual time, but do not give extra. Test again in four hours.
• greater than 13.0 mmol/L (over 230 mg/dL)	moderate or large	Give the usual insulin at the usual time. In addition, give, more of the superfast-acting or fast-acting insulin (10 to 20% of the total daily dose) *now*. Test again in four hours.

• greater than 17.0 mmol/L (300 mg/dL)	negative or small	Give the usual insulin at the usual time. In addition, give more of the superfast-acting or fast-acting (10 to 20% of the total daily dose) *now*. Test again in four hours.
• less than 6.0 mmol/L (110 mg/dL)	negative or positive	If it is time to give insulin, reduce the dose by 10 to 20%. Encourage consumption of sugar-containing fluids.

To figure out how much more fast-acting insulin to give, add up the total daily insulin dose. For example, someone taking 20 units of intermediate-acting and 4 units of fast-acting insulin before breakfast, 4 units of fast-acting insulin before supper and 7 units of intermediate-acting insulin before bed has a total of 35 units of insulin a day. Ten percent of 35 units is 3.5 units, and 20 percent of 35 units is 7 units, so give 4 to 7 units. Do not give more than 10 extra units at any one time. Small children tend to be sensitive so for them you should start with dosages at the lower end of the range.

Surgery

Most operations do not present problems for someone with diabetes, as long as careful attention is paid to blood sugar control before, during and after surgery.

Surgery under local anesthesia usually does not require hospital admission. However, it is important that meals not be missed. Dentists, for example, should be told about the diabetes, and appointments for tooth extraction or root canal work should be scheduled so they don't interfere with meal or snack times.

If surgery under general anesthetic is required, hospital admission may be necessary and a physician experienced in the management of Type 1 diabetes should be involved. Admission may be either one day before the surgery or on the day of surgery. On the day of surgery, an intravenous line will be used to supply fluids containing sugar until normal eating resumes. Also, the insulin dosage will be adjusted as necessary.

Q&A

I read that the symptoms of insulin reaction or diabetic ketoacidosis can be confused with drunkenness. Is that true?

It's true. The slurred speech, confusion, staggering and fatigue of hypoglycemia can look like drunken behavior. DKA may also be mistaken for drunkenness because the breath can smell a bit fruity, which can be confused with the smell of alcohol. However, what happens more often is that a person with diabetes has a couple of drinks, then begins to go low. (Alcohol causes low blood sugar if food isn't eaten at the same time.) A bystander who is unaware of the diabetes may smell alcohol on the breath and decide that the person is drunk. This is one good reason for someone with diabetes to wear a medical-alert bracelet.

My teenage son doesn't like to wear his medical-alert bracelet. How can I convince him it's the right thing to do?

While some children feel self-conscious about labeling themselves as having a special condition, these little medallions can be life-savers. Remind your son that the older he gets, the more time he will spend away from you, and with people who don't necessarily know he has diabetes. He needs to protect himself when you're not there.

Many young people find that wearing a medical-alert

bracelet can be an ice-breaker when they are unsure about raising the subject of diabetes. When new friends ask about the bracelet, they have the opportunity to explain, if they choose to do so.

How many insulin reactions are too many?
The occasional mild reaction, perhaps one or two per week, that can be easily treated with juice, is to be expected. However, these mild reactions can interrupt the school day or other activities, and make it difficult for the child to concentrate for the following half-hour or so. Prevent them as best you can, and respond to them quickly. Frequent lows need to be addressed with a change to the regimen. For example, if the teacher notices that your child is cranky every day at 11:30 a.m. and low blood sugar is confirmed, it's time to re-examine the meal plan or insulin dose and make a change.

What are the long-term effects of a severe low?
The greatest long-term effect is the fear that the child will have another severe insulin reaction. This is a very real fear for many parents, siblings and children with diabetes, and it can lead to a reluctance to keep trying to maintain good blood sugar control. This psychological setback is the only real long-term impact, because the body works very hard to protect the brain during events like this. In cases where diabetes started in infancy, some delayed intellectual development has been noted in infants who experienced repeated episodes of severe hypoglycemia in the first three to five years of life.

I heard that people sometimes smear honey in the mouth of a person with diabetes who is unable to swallow. Is this OK?
The big risk of giving an unconscious person anything by

mouth is that the person may choke on it. Smearing honey on the lips or between the gums and cheek of an unconscious person with diabetes is better than trying to pour juice or force a hard candy into the mouth. But using glucagon is the best way to reverse a severe hypoglycemic episode rapidly.

Is it possible to get diabetic ketoacidosis from eating too much sugar?
No. The worst that can happen is high blood sugar (hyperglycemia), which is undesirable but not the life-threatening condition of DKA. The only cause of DKA is a lack of insulin.

Is it all right to give my child cough syrup and other medicines?
If there is a cough syrup you find effective for your child, by all means use it as directed. The sugar content of the prescribed dose is probably minimal. However, if you're worried about the sugar in medications, ask your pharmacist to suggest preparations that are sugar-free.

Children with diabetes don't require medicine more than other children. However, if the doctor prescribes a course of antibiotics, for example, it's important to finish out the prescription, even if blood sugar levels begin to rise. Many parents mistakenly think the antibiotics are the cause of the blood glucose increase, but in fact the illness is probably causing stress on the body, leading to higher sugar levels.

There are medications containing steroids such as prednisone, sometimes prescribed for children with asthma, that actually do cause blood sugar to rise. These drugs can create a need for much more insulin, but they should not be withheld if they're needed. Be prepared to increase the insulin dose.

Should my child have a flu shot every year?
Children with diabetes do not get flu any more frequently or severely than their non-diabetic friends. However, when they do get sick the diabetes may be affected, as discussed. Having a flu shot may prevent your child from missing a few days of school and a period of upset in diabetes control. There is certainly no reason that children with diabetes should not have the flu shot or any other recommended immunizations.

Older children can treat mild reactions with dextrose tablets or hard candies. What would you suggest for infants and toddlers?
Clearly hard candies and dextrose tablets are inappropriate for young children. Three or four ounces (90–125 mL) of juice in a bottle or cup would work. Also, some parents keep a tube of cake frosting or other glucose-containing paste or gel handy for treating mild hypoglycemia.

S E V E N

Adjusting to Diabetes

S ometimes my folks and I seem to come from different planets," says Melissa, a 14-year-old who has had diabetes for the past eight years. "They seem to care only about my blood sugar numbers and not how I feel about myself. They don't trust me to take care of myself." Melissa's parents see it another way. "Melissa's a great kid, but left to her own devices, we're worried that she wouldn't test her sugars and might even skip a few insulin shots," says her mother, Joan. "It's so hard to let go after doing everything for her all these years, and she's not mature enough to make the right decisions on her own."

Melissa's situation is common among teenagers with diabetes. The struggle for independence versus the parents' reluctance to give up their caretaking role is one of the many phases of dealing with diabetes. From the day of diagnosis, diabetes has an immediate impact on the psychological, emotional and social functioning of the young person, as well as the family. Through the years, as the child or teen matures, the family faces many emotional challenges.

Dealing with the Diagnosis

The diagnosis of diabetes elicits many reactions in both child and parents. Most children and their families go through a grieving period at first, and experience a variety of feelings that may include shock, denial, sadness, anxiety, fear, anger and guilt. Over time, families do adjust and get on with life as they knew it; they find themselves adapting and readapting to diabetes, and feeling some of these emotions again and again.

Shock or Denial

"This can't be true!" When we experience a crisis our first reaction is often one of shock. This is our body's way of cushioning the blow. It's natural to feel numb and, early on, parents often say the reality hasn't hit them yet. Others describe the feeling as a bad dream from which they keep hoping to wake up. This feeling of shock is usually short-lived.

Sadness

"It feels like this is the end of the world." When we grieve, we feel a sense of loss or a deep sadness. Parents can feel shattered by the knowledge that their child has to receive injections, do blood tests and stick to a meal plan, and that these changes are likely permanent. Parents and children may mourn their old way of life. Children may be upset that they can't eat whenever they want to, or worry that it will affect their activities and friendships. Parents may feel bad that they have to say no sometimes to even "healthy food" because it isn't the right time of day to eat. Experiencing these emotions may help us begin to redefine our lives and put the pieces back together. Once people have expressed their sadness and sense of loss, they start to see the many parts of their lives, and the many hopes for their future, that don't have to change.

Fear and Anxiety

"How will we ever cope?" Confronted with diabetes and its implications, parents feel anxious about their child's health. Some worry about their ability to juggle the complex tasks required for good diabetes management, while others are more concerned about low blood sugar reactions. Some feel stressed about having to give injections or finger pricks. Still others worry about their child's future health, and wonder whether he or she will be able to manage alone in later years. Some children fear needle pricks or finger pricks in the beginning, and younger children, when they see their parents' distress, may even think they're going to die. However, their fear and anxiety often serve to focus the parents' attention on the needs of their children.

Anger and Resentment

"Why me?" Young people can be angry about developing diabetes. They may hate the injections, blood tests and food restrictions, and feel their world has turned upside down. They may feel it just isn't fair that they have to deal with this disease and its demands. Parents too can feel angry that this has happened, and helpless to change it. They may resent the extra responsibilities forced upon them. But anger can also empower parents in responding to and defending their children's needs.

Guilt

"What did we do wrong?" Parents often wonder if their child's diabetes is due to something they did, or blame themselves because diabetes runs in their family. Some feel guilty because they didn't notice the signs earlier. Children may feel they are burdening their parents. Some feel guilty, believing they must have done something wrong to cause the diabetes. There is absolutely no reason to feel guilty; there is nothing anyone can do to cause or prevent Type 1 diabetes. Guilt can be managed by refocusing on the things we do have some control over, such as treatment and future health.

All these difficult emotions can turn out to be positive and protective forces. But they can also be detrimental, if parents or children get stuck in one of these states. Talking about these early emotional reactions, and learning to manage them, helps families move along the path toward adjustment. During these early stages, the support of the diabetes team, including the social worker and psychologist or behavioral specialist, is very important. Their roles are not only to help stabilize the immediate medical condition, but also to provide support to the family.

Living with Diabetes

Adjusting takes time and patience for all family members. Everyone may have to get up a bit earlier on weekdays to accommodate the new routine; children may not be able to sleep in as late on weekends; parents will need to plan meals in advance instead of acting spontaneously (at first, anyway), and will have to remember to pack extra food for the child when he or she leaves the house. In the long run, though, all these adjustments become second nature.

Whenever possible, both parents should be involved in all phases of the diabetes care routine. Feelings of resentment, fatigue and stress can build up if one parent is burdened with all the planning and responsibility. Parents can work together to prevent "burnout" by sharing the load and giving each other time away from diabetes duties. They need to plan time together, apart from their child or children, just as they did before. The child will also benefit from growing up in a household where diabetes responsibilities are shared evenly.

In single-parent families, it helps if a member of the extended family or a close friend can participate in the child's care from time to time, or provide relief by babysitting. Take steps, though, to ensure that babysitters and other caregivers know enough about looking after a child with diabetes. Most diabetes teams will provide appropriate education for people participating in care at this level.

The challenge families face is to fit diabetes into their lifestyles, rather than letting it control their lives. This may require some creative problem-solving, often with help from the diabetes team. A strong support system of grandparents, aunts, uncles, siblings, friends and even support groups can do a lot to help you deal with the demands of diabetes, be it through practical or emotional support. Don't hesitate to ask for help from your diabetes team.

Attitudes and Beliefs

How families cope with diabetes depends to some extent on their attitudes and beliefs. Those who see it as a serious but manageable condition will cope better than those who remain overwhelmed, doubtful of their ability or negative about the potential long-term consequences of the disease. These attitudes and beliefs may be influenced by the family's prior experience with diabetes. Those who know someone having a difficult time, or experiencing serious complications, may feel very pessimistic about their own future. In this case, the diabetes team can help the family maintain perspective: science and technology have changed the outlook for people with this disorder, and there are positive steps you can take to decrease the chance of complications in later life.

Some parents view their child with diabetes as being sick or fragile at first. With a little time, education and experience they soon learn that their child is still healthy. They have to resist the urge to be overly concerned and overprotective, as this may interfere with the child's normal development. Diabetes should not stop children and teens from doing all the things their friends would do. It's just that extra planning is needed to ensure their safety.

Balancing Supervision with Independence

Diabetes requires that both the young person and the parents acquire new skills and take on new tasks. These added responsibilities inevitably alter family relationships. With very young children, total responsibility for all aspects of day-to-day activities will fall squarely on the parents. However, as the child grows and matures there will be a slow and steady shift from completely parent-oriented care, through stages of shared care, to complete independence of the late adolescent and young adult in all aspects of diabetes management.

The transfer of responsibility must not be too rapid. New responsibilities should be added only as the child or teen demonstrates competence with those parts of the treatment plan he or she is already responsible for. The teens who run into the most difficulty with their diabetes are those for whom parental support is either lacking or inconsistent. Some health care providers mistakenly encourage families to give as much responsibility as possible to the child. After all, they argue, it's the child's diabetes and the child must become proficient in its management. The best balance, however, requires that parents continue to support and encourage their teens, to help them achieve and maintain the best possible level of glucose control. Parents obviously walk a thin line between giving too much responsibility too early and being overprotective. That's one reason the diabetes team is there to guide them.

Even when a young teen has been responsible for a good deal of diabetes care without much supervision, the parents will need to become more involved when the going gets tough, such as during periods of illness, stress at school or other emotional crises.

Emotional Impact on Brothers and Sisters

Siblings go through the same emotions as other family members: guilt that their brother or sister has diabetes and they haven't; fear that they too may get the disease, or that their sibling may become really sick; anger that Mom or Dad stopped buying sugar-coated cereals or baking chocolate chip muffins; jealousy because their sibling seems to get all the attention. It's a challenge, especially at the time of diagnosis, to balance everyone's needs. Brothers and sisters need to be given the opportunity to express their feelings and emotions, and to know that they are still loved. They should be encouraged to participate in the education program, both to involve them in the new family reality and to provide information that will allow them to feel safe and comfortable with their sibling with diabetes. Many parents find that spending "special time" alone with non-diabetic siblings eases the emotional impact on them.

Financial Concerns

The ongoing cost of diabetes supplies can be a concern. The child requires insulin, syringes or pen injectors and needles; blood sugar monitoring equipment (meters and strips); urine test strips; glucagon emergency kits; glucose tablets for low sugar reactions. Clearly diabetes is an expensive disease: for example, blood sugar test strips cost eighty cents to a dollar (both U.S. and Canadian) each. For someone checking blood glucose levels three or four times a day, this can add up to a considerable amount of money every year, for the strips alone. Most drug plans cover the cost of most diabetes supplies. For those who have no coverage and cannot afford these supplies, federal or provincial/state plans may help alleviate the burden. Volunteer agencies may also provide financial support. But some families have to pay for diabetes supplies themselves, because they don't have private insurance and they aren't eligible for government plans. This can be quite a hefty load. At the very least, these expenses should be eligible for a medical expense tax credit. If you're in this position, ask your diabetes team about agencies, resources and strategies that may help ease the financial load.

Impact of the Family and Child on the Diabetes

Just as diabetes impacts on the family, so the way the family functions affects diabetes management. A healthy adjustment tends to be associated with family sharing of responsibilities, feelings of family togetherness, the ability to problem-solve, little conflict between family members and consistent child management. When there is overwhelming stress in the family, it's hard to think through problems and solve them effectively. As a result, diabetes care may be compromised.

Healthy attitudes in the parents are key to helping children adjust; children take their cues from their parents and are sensitive to their feelings. When parents are consistent in their expectations and agree on the approach to diabetes management, the child is more likely to comply with routines. It also helps if parents are used to problem-solving and have developed coping strategies around stress in their own lives.

Diabetes and Friends

Childhood and adolescence are periods of frequent and intense social interaction. While parents are trying to figure out how to deal with daily diabetes management, young people are often more worried about how to incorporate this new reality into their lives. Plenty of questions arise: What do I tell my friends? How do I tell them? Will they treat me differently now that I have to take daily injections, check my blood sugar and eat my meals at specific times? Just as each family has different ways of coping with diabetes in general, children and teens have different styles of telling their friends.

With a little encouragement, most children will choose an open, matter-of-fact approach. Often they make a presentation on diabetes to the class as part of "show-and-tell." Some choose to share their experience and knowledge as part of a science project. Most classmates are curious, and full of admiration for a friend who is brave enough to endure daily injections and finger pricks.

But not all children are comfortable with this approach. Some hesitate to discuss their diabetes with classmates they hardly know. Rather, they prefer to share the information only with school personnel and their closest friends, the ones they rely on for support. For safety's sake, the families of the child's friends should also be aware of the diabetes, the need for routines and even the signs and symptoms of a low blood glucose reaction.

Some children would prefer to hide their diabetes. This is unsafe and may even be psychologically unhealthy, reflecting unresolved denial or shame. A child who is not prepared to tell friends about his or her diabetes may have poor self-esteem and a lack of confidence. While respecting the child's wish for privacy, parents may have to help the child share the diagnosis with close friends, key school personnel and other caregivers to ensure a safe environment.

One reason children want to avoid telling their friends is the fear of teasing or shunning. Fortunately, teasing is not that common. If teasing is an issue, children may need some special tips and support in handling the situation.

The family, the school and the diabetes team can all play a supportive role in helping the child talk to friends and deal with their varied reactions. Parents can speak to the friends' parents and help the child feel more self-confident. The school can explain to classmates that diabetes is not contagious, and that the child with diabetes is no different from other children and can continue to enjoy the same games and activities as before. Among the members of the diabetes team, the social worker or counselor is usually best equipped to deal with these coping issues, recognizing children's varied backgrounds, personal experiences and family dynamics.

Strategies for Adjustment

In addition to the usual varied stresses most families face, families living with diabetes face additional demands. How can they ease the burden and adjust to the disease as smoothly as possible?

- *Learn as much as possible about diabetes.* Becoming an expert means you'll more likely be ready when a challenge arises.
- *Keep in regular contact with the diabetes team.* These health professionals are there to help with problem-solving. Sometimes a call to one of the team can quickly solve a problem that seems insurmountable. Don't let a small problem grow.
- *Explore community and social supports.* Knowing other families who have a child with diabetes, belonging to a

parent support group or, for teens themselves, joining a diabetes youth group may lessen the tension by providing the opportunity to meet understanding peers.

- *Share the responsibility.* In two-parent families, find an appropriate balance of responsibilities and activities related to diabetes care. Single parents should try to find a support person who is willing to learn the basics about the child's diabetes routines and to provide necessary relief. With this back-up in place, the child remains safe when the parent is not available.

- *Remember what worked before to relieve stress.* Fall back on familiar ways of coping that have worked in the past. This may involve taking time out, going for a walk, talking with a friend, listening to music or enjoying a vigorous physical workout.

- *Manage feelings—don't hide them.* Although it is often hard for parents to see their children upset, it is important to allow them to express painful feelings about having diabetes. This helps children feel understood and supported, and parents feel relieved knowing what the problem is. Solid communication builds trust and promotes problem-solving, important factors in healthy adjustment to a chronic disorder.

- *Use distractions.* For the small child, in particular, the actual performance of blood sugar checks and insulin injections may cause tension. Have the child hold a teddy bear during the injection, perform the finger pricks while the child watches television or have a sibling sit with the child while the routines are completed.

- *Try not to focus only on the diabetes.* Remember that children lead busy and active lives. Make an effort to focus on their schoolwork, their friends or their extracurricular activities. Get involved in these activities in a way that's consistent with your lifestyle, and demonstrate by your action and interest that diabetes is not your only shared activity.

- *Avoid black and white thinking.* Diabetes care can be complicated, and it's important not to think of outcomes as good or bad. Blood glucose and HbA_{1c} levels should be thought of as high or low, not good or bad. Furthermore, diabetes care is not an "all or nothing" issue. Viewing temporary problems as slips, not failures, will make adapting easier.

Diabetes in the Classroom

The demands of diabetes management cannot help but have an impact on school life. School personnel must be aware of the student with diabetes. By understanding the important aspects of diabetes management, the teacher can ensure the student's healthy adjustment to the classroom setting and peer interactions. Teachers also play an important part in ensuring the safety of the student with diabetes, not only in the classroom but in the playground, on school trips and in sports activities. A knowledgeable and supportive teacher will help allay parental anxiety, and will prevent minor crises from getting out of hand. A poorly informed or misinformed teacher who has great anxiety about having a student with diabetes in the classroom can add to the adjustment and management difficulties encountered by the child and the family.

To avert potential problems, arrange a meeting with the child's teachers and other school personnel at the beginning of the school year (or soon after diagnosis, if that happens during the school year) to discuss the child's individual needs.

General health care is the responsibility of the family, with the help of the diabetes team. Teachers and other school personnel (excluding the school nurse) are not health care professionals, but they do have a role to play in supporting students and ensuring their safety. It is unrealistic to expect the majority of teachers to be well informed about every disorder that a student may someday show up with. However, when a student with a disorder does arrive in their classroom, teachers and school personnel should gain the necessary know-how to provide support. How much participation is expected from teachers will depend on the child's age, stage of development and diabetes routines.

The most important thing for teachers to know about diabetes is how to recognize hypoglycemia and prevent a mild insulin reaction from escalating into a more severe one. Teachers of younger children need to be especially observant during gym periods, and remind the child with diabetes to take a snack. Teachers should also understand that meal plans are an important element of diabetes care, and that it's hard for children with diabetes to participate in surprise pizza parties or snacks. Teachers should inform parents of any such events so they can adjust the child's meal plan accordingly. They should be aware of the need for between-meal snacks. Similarly, they should become familiar with the signs of hyperglycemia, and notify parents if the child has to leave the classroom to go to the bathroom more frequently than usual.

In general, teachers should not be expected or required to perform blood sugar checks or inject insulin. If these become necessary, the teacher should be properly educated to ensure safe and effective management. The school should have a plan of action in place in case the child has a severe insulin reaction: administer sugar or juice if the child is conscious; if unconscious, call an ambulance. If the child vomits, the parents or some other designated, responsible adult should be notified. If they are unavailable, the teacher must get the child to the nearest emergency room.

Keeping the school informed

When completed, this form contains the information parents need to provide to teachers and school personnel at the beginning of each school year. The information should be updated as necessary.

Student's name _____ Age _____ Grade _____

Parents' names_____

Address _____

Phone: home _____Business _____Cell/pager _____

Alternate person to call in an emergency_____

Phone_____

Are there siblings in school? Yes _____No _____

   Names _____Grades _____

Doctor's name _____Phone_____

Health insurance number _____

Time(s) of day when an insulin (hypoglycemic) reaction may occur:

_____

Symptoms commonly experienced by the student: _____

_____

What has been provided to treat the reactions:_____

_____

Where is this sugar source located? _____

   alternatives   4 oz (125 mL) fruit juice
                   4 oz (125 mL) regular soft drink (not diet)

Type of morning snack_____

Type of afternoon snack _____

Suggested treats for in-school parties_____

Suggested food for extra activities _____

Special instructions _____

_____

_____   [photo of
_____   child goes
_____   here]
_____

_____

Field Trips

Children with diabetes should be encouraged to participate in as many school activities as they choose, and should not be excluded from school trips. However, planning ahead is essential. If they are participating in physical activities beyond those they do on a daily basis, extra food should be packed in their knapsack or lunch box. Include a mix of fast-acting carbohydrate snacks, such as juice boxes and dried fruit to stave off low sugar reactions, and complex carbohydrate snacks such as crackers, breakfast bars and cookies.

Careful preparation for overnight trips or special events will help prevent problems. If the event—for example, a field trip to the zoo—overlaps an insulin injection or blood test time, ensure that one of the teachers or chaperoning parents is taking responsibility for either performing or supervising the task. Children and accompanying adults should always have supplies to treat low blood sugar, such as hard candies, glucose gels—even a glucagon kit for overnight or longer trips, if a responsible adult is taught how to use it. Children should know how to recognize symptoms of low blood sugar before they are permitted to go on overnight field trips. Before that, look at volunteering as a chaperone yourself.

What to pack on a field trip

On field trips of any type, the child with diabetes must have:

- a source of quick-fix concentrated carbohydrate to treat hypoglycemia (i.e. juice boxes, glucose tablets, hard candies)
- visible identification that indicates that the student has diabetes, such as a medical-alert bracelet
- insulin, syringes and blood testing equipment, if the trip overlaps a testing or injection time
- an informed adult companion
- the phone number of parents or an alternate, well-informed responsible adult

Summer Camp

For many school-age children and teens, summertime means not only a holiday from school, but also the opportunity to play and spend time with friends at either day camps or overnight residential camps. For children with diabetes the situation is no different, and with proper planning they too can enjoy a fun-filled, healthy and safe camp experience. The preparation for day camps is similar to preparation for a family day out or a day trip at school. Make sure the child has all meals and snacks prepared and packed. Except for children who are on a lunchtime injection and are able to administer it themselves, with minor adjustments in timing all insulin injections can be given at home as usual. Similarly, at least three daily blood glucose tests can be performed at home, and blood glucose levels can be monitored by a parent. Most children should do a pre-lunch glucose check at camp.

Ask camp staff about the level of activity in which the child will participate. Inform them that the child has diabetes and emphasize the importance of the timing of food intake. The signs and symptoms of hypoglycemia should be explained, and a source of rapid-acting sugar should be supplied to a counselor to treat a low blood glucose reaction. Furthermore, the camp staff must, like teachers, be told what to do in the event of a severe insulin reaction.

What about residential camps? Are they safe for children with diabetes? Absolutely. However, to provide a happy and safe camping experience and to ensure that the principles of daily diabetes care are followed, many diabetes organizations have set up camps especially for children with diabetes. Whenever possible, children and teens with diabetes should have the chance to attend such camps. They are usually staffed by doctors and nurses experienced in the care of children with diabetes. In addition, an experienced dietitian is there to develop the child's individual meal plan and adjust it during the camping period. The programming staff are accustomed to working with campers with diabetes, and develop programs to match the timing of daily diabetes routines. These camps give children the opportunity to spend several days or weeks with other campers who also have diabetes.

Having spent most of the school year integrated with children who do not, many campers are excited to be with other campers who are going through the same stages of disease management. Everybody is doing blood checks, testing urine, taking insulin injections, monitoring diet and watching for low blood sugar reactions. Some children learn to give their own injections for the first time under the direction of the camp nurse and with the encouragement of their summer friends. For others, especially those from smaller communities, this may be their first experience of not being the only child with diabetes.

Children aren't the only ones who benefit from camp. Many parents find comfort in knowing that diabetes routines are being followed and that their children are in the care of competent staff familiar with the disease, whether at the campsite or during multi-day canoe trips. They feel secure in the knowledge that blood glucose checks will be done overnight as necessary, as well as during the day, and that extra snacks will be provided when needed. With such a support system, the children can enjoy the full range of camp experiences, including swimming, boating, tripping, crafts and drama, without the burden of managing their diabetes care alone.

Some teens prefer to go to residential camps not specifically aimed at those with diabetes. If the teen has sufficient knowledge, sense of responsibility and willingness to monitor the condition, this too can be accommodated by proper planning. The teen becomes more responsible for sticking to the meal plan, monitoring blood glucose and adjusting insulin doses.

Remember that most children attending camp are more active than usual, and have less access to food between meals. As a result, they may require a lower or different insulin dose to avoid hypoglycemic episodes. More frequent blood glucose monitoring will be needed to determine the actual insulin requirement. Whenever possible, choose a camp with a full-time physician and nurse on site, who can help deal with diabetes routines and any illness that may occur.

Letting Go

The day will come when the child with diabetes is no longer living under the family roof. This transition can be traumatic for both child and parent. No longer will the parent be able to monitor the child's daily log of insulin doses and glucose readings. Nor will the parent be around to pick up on the child's trademark symptoms of an insulin reaction. The solution? Start laying a foundation for independence early on. Encourage and support age-appropriate involvement of your child in his or her own diabetes care.

Q&A

Will we ever take a vacation alone again?
It may take a while before you feel comfortable enough with your child's diabetes care to leave someone else in charge. But sooner or later you will. And it's important that you do so, to avoid burnout. You can ease the anxiety by starting off gradually, with a short trip a couple of hours' drive away (you'll feel better knowing you can return home quickly), rather than a two-week vacation in South America. If you know, for example,

that you have a week-long business trip you can't miss, you can prepare yourself in advance by spending a night with friends or relatives. Giving a sitter this kind of "dry run" may also alleviate his or her concerns, as well as the concerns of your child. Give your sitter and any siblings the telephone numbers of your diabetes health care team (and alert the team that they may be called by someone other than yourself). Provide relevant reading material and make up a diabetes care instruction sheet specific to your child.

People keep telling me I should join a diabetes support group, but I'm not sure if they're for me. What are they all about?
Support groups can be invaluable sources of information and advice and, in many cases, new friendships. Your diabetes team or local diabetes association can provide names of group leaders. If there is no support group in your area, you may want to start your own. Support groups meet on a regular basis— some follow formal agendas, while others are casual social gatherings. There is little, if any, cost involved, and you're not obligated to attend every meeting.

Some people resist support groups because they don't like the idea of identifying themselves as "afflicted." But in some ways support groups free you from this label, because everyone there knows the road you are traveling. You don't have to explain the biology and psychology of diabetes to get to the point of your problem. Sharing experiences provides a way to learn more about diabetes, and to feel more secure about your effectiveness in dealing with it.

How can I convince my parents that they don't need to worry about me anymore?
Parents will always worry about their children. But you can

help them worry less by showing them that you are sensible in managing your diabetes, and that you make good decisions in other areas of your life.

Every time Billy's grandparents come to visit, they shower him with chocolate and candy. How can we make them see this is harmful for Billy?
It's natural for grandparents to want to give gifts to their grandchildren. You may want to encourage them to pamper Billy in other ways, such as with trips to the movies, or snacks like popcorn or chips. When the gifts are food, help Billy accept them graciously, and then help him work the treat into his meal plan.

My brother keeps telling me he wishes he had diabetes. Why would he say that?
Believe it or not, your brother is probably jealous of the attention you receive. This is normal, but if his comments make you uncomfortable, tell him you don't like him saying that, and tell him how you feel about having diabetes. Your brother may also be sad that you have to deal with diabetes, and may wish you weren't going through this. It's a good idea to talk to your parents too, so everyone understands how everyone else is feeling.

Our daughter does well in school but often complains of headaches or stomach cramps due to anxiety about going to school in the morning. What does this mean?
Your daughter may be experiencing school avoidance, which occurs commonly in children with a chronic condition such as diabetes. There are many reasons why children may become anxious. In a child with diabetes, the avoidance may have to do with being teased, or with fear of having a low reaction.

Take time to explore your daughter's fears and anxieties about school and diabetes, and seek help from your diabetes team.

The children at my son's school keep teasing him about his diabetes. What should I do?

We can all remember being teased about something at some stage of our childhood—wearing glasses, having skinny legs, even just bringing something unusual for lunch! Diabetes can be one more target for teasing, but the subject may be a particularly sensitive one, not only for your son but for you as well. It's important to recognize your own vulnerability here, so that you can put the teasing in perspective and work with your son to generate some creative solutions.

An impromptu family discussion about how to handle teasing and the teasers often helps give the child some ideas, as well as moral support. Some children learn to use humor as a response. For others, knowledge is power. It allows them to deal confidently with their classmates' misconceptions, and gains them respect for coping with the disease.

If you believe the teasing results from ignorance, you and your son may want to talk to his teacher about strategies to help his classmates understand the basics of diabetes, and what it means to live with it.

EIGHT

Growth and Development

Lisa is a typical 12-year-old—her three best friends are the most important thing in her life. The four of them spend almost every waking hour together, talking about boys, trying new hairstyles, turning cartwheels in the backyard. Lisa likes her friends and cares what they think. They know she has diabetes and she doesn't want them to think for one minute that it means she can't do everything they can. This is a good attitude on Lisa's part, but it could get her into trouble if it prevents her from sticking to her diabetes routines. For instance, one day after school Lisa was so caught up in hanging out with her friends that she forgot she needed to get home for her afternoon snack. By 4:30 she felt shaky, hungry and a little dizzy. Fortunately one of her friends had a little candy which she gave Lisa, and after a few minutes Lisa felt better. Of course, Lisa's mom was upset when she found out, but she understood Lisa's wanting to stay with her friends. So they made a deal: from now on Lisa will always carry an extra snack with her, in case she's going to be late.

Each age and stage of life presents a different set of challenges relating to both physical and emotional growth and development. A chronic disorder brings additional challenges. It seems that, as soon as the family has found ways to negotiate the rocky course of one stage of development, it's time to go to the next stage. For example, parenting a school-age child with diabetes can be much different from parenting an infant or toddler. Likewise, being a teenager with diabetes is different from being nine or ten and living with the disorder. As teenagers reach adulthood, they are faced with new issues that further affect their diabetes care.

The family and the diabetes team can both help smooth the road to adulthood by promoting a strong sense of identity and self-worth in the growing child. The best predictor of future behavior is past behavior: a child whose course has been relatively smooth throughout early childhood is quite likely to negotiate adolescence successfully. Also, families that provide age-appropriate support and guidance will no doubt have less disruption to deal with during the teen years.

Infants, Toddlers and Preschoolers

Type 1 diabetes is less common in preschoolers than in older children and adolescents: less than 1 percent of diabetes is diagnosed in the first year of life, and less than 10 percent before the age of five. Because diabetes is uncommon in this age group and because the symptoms are often confused with other minor illnesses, the diagnosis is often missed until the baby is very sick, in severe diabetic ketoacidosis. Once the disease is diagnosed, however, the situation can be corrected quickly and long-term management can begin.

Developmental milestones and patterns affect the very young child's perception of the world. Normal infants and toddlers generally:

- determine thoughts by what they see and hear
- begin to develop a sense of themselves, first by acquiring a trust in their environment as infants, and then by testing this environment in the next few years
- enhance their knowledge of the world around them through constant exploration, language development and inquiry ("Why this? Why that? Why the other thing?")
- begin to become more curious and self-directed, choosing some activities and rejecting others

Diabetes care in children under five involves a balance between what might be considered ideal—close to normal blood sugar readings—and what is safe and practical. The target range for these young children—pre-meal sugars of 6–12 mmol/L (110–220 mg/dL)—allows good blood glucose control while reducing the risk of severe hypoglycemia. Too tight control in infants and toddlers is especially risky as they cannot yet recognize the symptoms of low blood sugar. Repeated episodes of severe hypoglycemia in these children may lead to mild intellectual or learning impairment later in life.

Very young children often have fluctuating appetites. They don't always eat the same amount of food from day to day. If pre-meal blood sugar levels are allowed to go slightly higher than what might be expected for older children, the infant or toddler is more likely to remain safe even during periods of food refusal or picky eating. Parents will be less worried and frustrated and mealtime will be more pleasant. As children grow they become more predictable in their eating, and more able to recognize and describe their low blood sugar reactions. At that time blood sugar targets also change.

Signs of a Healthy Infant or Toddler with Diabetes
How do parents and others who care for young children know that everything is going well? Look for:
- normal growth and weight gain
- developmental milestones, such as rolling over, sitting up, crawling, standing, walking and talking, at about the normal age
- no signs of high blood sugar levels; good energy, not overly wet (diapers) or unusually thirsty
- few mild low blood sugar reactions, and no severe reactions
- no ketones in the urine
- blood sugar readings that are not too low—less than 6.0 mmol/L (110 mg/dL)
- blood sugar readings that are not too high for long periods of time—over 12 mmol/L (220 mg/dL)
- a happy and secure attitude in the child

Impact of Diabetes on an Infant, Toddler or Preschooler
Young children with Type 1 diabetes progress through the same stages of development as their friends without diabetes. Nevertheless, the routines and tasks needed for good diabetes care may influence and sometimes interfere with this development. All parents of young children with diabetes worry about the effects of diabetes on their growth as individuals, and how they will cope with the condition as they grow older.
Specific areas of concern include:
- the young child's inability to express symptoms of hypoglycemia (e.g., is the toddler having a hypoglycemic spell or a temper tantrum?)
- dealing with their own and their child's anxiety about the pricks and injections
- developing a structured but flexible treatment plan that

does not interfere with the child's normal daily activities, including naps
• providing meals and snacks on time and in consistent amounts (those picky toddlers can really cause stress at mealtimes)

Try to balance the child's need for support and protection against the risk of overprotection and exclusion from age-appropriate activities.

Eating habits change rapidly during the first five years of life. Some infants and toddlers are relatively consistent in their eating patterns; most, however, have wide fluctuations in appetite and the amount of food they eat. It's important that the diabetes care routine reflect that. For safety's sake, young children should eat at regular meal and snack times—at least three meals and three snacks a day. But imposing a highly structured meal plan on an infant or toddler may only heighten the stress in the family, and even interfere with the child's normal development. As the child gets older, more structure in meal planning becomes both possible and necessary.

Coping Strategies
Some helpful hints in coping with diabetes in a young child include:
• Try to adopt a matter-of-fact approach to insulin injections, finger pricks and mealtimes. Young children quickly pick up on parents' anxieties and use them to manipulate their environment. Try to be quick, calm and reassuring when carrying out routines. Reduce the child's fears by preparing the insulin or blood testing equipment in another room before involving the child. When it's over, give the child a big hug and a kiss.

- Share responsibility for the routines wherever possible. In single-parent families, have a friend or family member participate in the diabetes routines on a regular basis. This prevents the toddler from playing one caregiver off against the other. The parent, the toddler and the support person can remain confident that the child will be safe in the parent's absence.
- Acknowledge the child's feelings and provide reassurance, but don't delay needles or finger pricks until the child is "ready." Consider using distractions such as toys, songs or television.
- Try to allow the child some control over the routine if he or she wishes: for example, choosing the finger for the next prick.
- For the really picky eater, set limits on time allowed for meals and snacks. Don't sit for hours fighting over each morsel of food. The child always wins.

Tommy is two and a half, and doing quite well with his diabetes routines. His parents, Heather and Marc, are sharing responsibility for his finger pricks and insulin injections. Heather gives the morning shot and Marc does the second one, before the evening meal. Tommy's four-year-old brother, Tyler, is usually asleep during Tommy's morning routine— which suits Heather just fine—but Tyler likes to help his dad with the evening blood sugar check and insulin shot, leaving Heather free to get dinner on the table. Meal and snack times are consistent. Both boys enjoy settling in for their morning snack just as their favorite television program starts at 10 a.m. Afternoon snack works equally well, following Tommy's nap, at 3 p.m. The only problem for Heather comes when Tommy sleeps past 3 p.m. She hates to wake him, figuring he must need his sleep, but how long can she safely let him nap? Unlike children without diabetes, he can't nap right through his snack time. She decides, with the help of her diabetes team, that an extra half-hour is the limit.

Lately Tommy has been refusing food, especially at mealtimes. Worried about lows, Heather and Marc have been pleading, coaxing and even preparing two or three food choices, but in the end Tommy holds out for apple juice. After discussion with the diabetes team, Heather and Marc decide to reduce the insulin dose a little and adjust the blood sugar targets to 8–12 mmol/L (145–220 mg/dL), from 6–12 mmol/L (110–220 mg/dL), to allow for food refusal, and to limit mealtime to a maximum of 25 minutes. They also plan to resist, if possible, replacing the meal with apple juice alone. Food refusal is a temporary stage many toddlers go through. As Tommy's appetite becomes more predictable, they will have to increase the insulin and reset the blood sugar targets.

The School-aged Child

Starting school is an exciting time for both child and parents. Children will spend a major part of their day away from home, away from the parents' watchful eye. Not until late childhood or early adolescence can the child be expected to understand diabetes treatment fully, and integrate all its important concepts, such as timing and amounts of insulin injections, blood sugar checks, and consistency in eating habits.

Normal developmental patterns in the early school years include:

- learning to solve concrete problems logically
- further development of social skills—the peer group begins to take on more importance
- learning to play by the rules and thrive in a structured and

supportive environment; when children know the rules and can acquire appropriate skills in a fun way, they develop a positive self-image
- learning to conform

Impact of Diabetes on School-aged Children

Parents usually continue to be the predominant caregivers, but they are more frequently required to share expertise not only with the child but with other responsible people such as teachers, sports coaches, babysitters and day care staff.

School-aged children may see themselves as different from their peers, which can lead to considerable distress. Classmates may tease them about their needles and finger pricks. Be sure the child has an appropriate understanding of diabetes, but encourage him or her to participate in school and other activities in the same way other children do. Naturally, planning is required, but being excluded from these activities can be detrimental to the child's self-image.

Coping Strategies

- Remain actively involved in all aspects of your child's diabetes care throughout childhood. However, the level and type of your involvement will change as the child participates more and more in the routines. Ongoing parental involvement in a supportive and nonjudgmental manner will help the child overcome hurdles along the way.
- Be prepared for the occasional slip-up. As children assume more responsibility, they make mistakes—eating a little more, skipping a snack, recording a false blood sugar reading, perhaps even missing an injection. These lapses are a normal part of growing up. Expect them and watch for them so you can deal with them before there are any serious

consequences. But remember that these lapses are not a sign of failure. Rather, they provide an opportunity to talk about diabetes and its challenges, and to open the door to creative problem-solving.

• Establish routines, such as mealtime and snack time, and stick to these when possible. However, flexibility is key. Don't fret over a change in schedule, but be aware of the adjustments to be made when, for example, a meal or snack is delayed, or an insulin injection is scheduled during a sports event.

• Involve the child in the routines, and acknowledge his or her feelings and concerns about diabetes. Encourage children's mastery of the diabetes routines—choosing snacks, doing finger pricks and insulin injections.

• Children should be encouraged and helped, rather than forced or threatened, to get them to comply with routines. Opt for simple reminders rather than long lectures.

• Try to control your own stresses, frustrations and anxieties surrounding diabetes. Children are sensitive to these displays and may either mirror your responses, or try to hide things from you to avoid upsetting you. Seek support from the diabetes team, other parents of children with diabetes or a support group.

Susan is ten years old and has had diabetes since age four. Her parents take most of the responsibility for her diabetes but Susan does help out. She has been able to do her own finger pricks and blood checks for a couple of years now, but must be reminded *when* to do them. Her parents record the results. Susan is pretty good at choosing the right kinds and amounts of food at mealtimes and snack times. She knows what it feels like to be low, and she knows what to do—take three dextrose tablets. She hasn't yet mastered her insulin injection—she just hasn't been interested, and her parents have been willing to stay in charge. But Susan is in grade five now and her class will be going to an outdoor education camp for three days. Susan is determined to go too. Her parents are anxious and want to say no—but instead, knowing they have several months to prepare, they sit down with Susan and their diabetes nurse and come up with a plan that will prepare the family and the teacher for this adventure.

Because there may not be an adult on the school trip who can prepare and inject insulin safely, Susan's parents agree to work with her over the next few months to ensure that she is confident and competent with insulin injections by the time she's ready to go.

Susan is already able to do her blood glucose and urine ketone checks, so the next step is for her to begin entering results in the record book for practice one week a month. Susan thinks this is a good idea.

Because she already makes good decisions about food choices every day, Susan's parents will begin to involve her in planning for extra activity with extra food.

Finally, Susan's mother will contact those at the school in charge of organizing the outdoor camp to find out about adult supervision, the program of activity, the meal schedule and opportunities for communication between Susan and her parents during camp. She will also organize an education session with the adult taking primary responsibility for Susan at camp. This person must remind Susan about testing and insulin injection times, supervise these routines and, if necessary, help her respond to low blood glucose or get in touch with her family. These are not unrealistic expectations of an adult supervisor of a grade five student.

Adolescence

Adolescence is a time of rapid biological change, accompanied by increasing physical, cognitive and emotional maturity. It is a time of increasing peer conformity, experimentation, limit-testing and independence from family. Self-image changes with the emergence of sexuality, and the experience may be difficult and even frightening for some. Diabetes can affect these processes in different ways.

With or without diabetes, the progression of adolescent development varies greatly both across and within age groups, and within individuals. An important milestone is the acquisition of abstract reasoning, which allows the adolescent to understand fully the implications of diabetes and its management. There are, however, many compelling and conflicting factors—peer pressure, parties and other social events, part-time jobs and a busy life in general—that may interfere with the teen's ability to translate this new awareness into good self-care behaviors.

Normal developmental patterns during adolescence

Early adolescence (12–14)
- places enormous importance on body image and is intensely self-absorbed
- seeks reassurance more and more from peers rather than family

Mid-adolescence (14–17)
- struggles for autonomy and control of personal destiny
- can be involved in teen-parent conflict, centering on relatively trivial issues such as hair length, clothes and curfew, as well as more serious issues such as smoking, alcohol and drug use
- may indulge in other risk-taking behaviors

Late adolescence (18–21)
- becomes increasingly stable (true of many but not all teens)
- begins to shape long-term plans such as career and personal goals

Even though it may seem that these young people should be more responsible, more able to achieve "good" blood sugar control, adolescence is frequently the time when adequate blood sugar control is most difficult.

Impact of Diabetes on Adolescents

Diabetes management requires a degree of responsibility and behavioral control that is uncharacteristic of adolescents. The daily demands of the disease have an impact on the personal and public lives of these teens, affecting important developmental areas including independence, body image, identity, sexuality, responsibility and self-esteem. Parents worry a lot about the teenage years, and perhaps more so when their teen has diabetes. Yet recent research suggests that most adolescents navigate this period without too much disruption, and that they are, in fact, quite well adjusted.

Coping Strategies

- Remain involved in your child's diabetes care, at some level, right through adolescence. Diabetes management is a heavy burden to carry alone.
- Let go gradually. Make sure your teen is ready, willing and able to take on the aspects of diabetes management you are ready to give up.
- Praise adolescents freely. There is no danger of giving them an inflated ego, and positive reinforcement will only yield more of the desired behavior.
- Parents, teens and the diabetes team must all have the same expectations of the teen and of each other. Is everyone aiming for the same blood sugar targets? Can everyone agree on the frequency of blood glucose monitoring? Can everyone agree about who chooses what foods at mealtime? Goals

and expectations should be reviewed jointly, on a regular basis, to be sure they're still appropriate.

• All teens hate to be nagged, but most don't mind a little help. Parents can help get the monitoring equipment ready for a check, instead of simply saying, "It's that time again." Similarly, they can offer to keep the log, instead of complaining that they don't know what's going on because the numbers never get into the book.

• Be prepared to get reinvolved as necessary. Even the most self-sufficient teen is going to need back-up during particularly stressful periods, such as a crisis in a relationship, an illness or a time of overwhelming competing priorities. This is not a step backward; it's just evidence of the family working together to ensure that the teen's health is maintained at all times.

• Teens should be encouraged to develop their own relationships with members of their diabetes team. Allow a teen private time with the doctor or nurse at each clinic visit. It's natural for parents to want to stay informed, and to have time to discuss issues and be part of developing the plan for the next phase. However, teens should be able to expect confidentiality in certain aspects of their health care.

Special Considerations in the Teenaged Years

Smoking, drug and alcohol abuse in both teenaged boys and girls, and unplanned pregnancies and eating disorders in girls, are common hazards. However, teens with diabetes must be fully aware of the problems associated with these behaviors, and the additional risks to their health. The use of alcohol, for example, increases the risk of severe hypoglycemia, and smoking greatly increases the chance of early stroke, heart attack and other diabetes-related complications. It is impossible to make wise choices without accurate information.

It is also critical for parents to understand that diabetes routines may become a target for risk-taking behavior. Teens may skip meals or blood sugar checks. Some even skip their insulin. If such behavior seriously compromises diabetes control, resulting in poor school attendance, hospitalization (due to diabetic ketoacidosis) or poor growth or weight loss, parents will need to resume giving the injections and doing the blood sugar checks, regardless of the teen's age, until there is evidence that it's safe to allow the teen to manage independently once again.

Smoking and Drug Use

Many teens try cigarettes. Unfortunately, some become regular users. Experimenting with "street drugs" such as marijuana is also not uncommon. Adolescents try out tobacco and drugs for several reasons: peer pressure, risk-taking and feeling "grown up," relief from stress, or because the family does.

Smoking dramatically increases the risk of serious diabetes-related complications such as eye and kidney disease, early stroke and heart attacks. It should be avoided at all costs. Parents, coaches, educators and health care providers should make sure children know the risks of smoking from a very young age, and should do whatever it takes to discourage the habit. For parents, this may mean giving up smoking themselves. Teens who have already started smoking may benefit from a smoking cessation program offered at school or perhaps at an adolescent medicine clinic or public health unit.

Marijuana impairs the judgment required to recognize and acknowledge the signs of low blood sugar. Marijuana use also triggers food cravings and hunger, leading to overeating which can, in turn, cause high blood sugar. The direct effect of other "street drugs" on blood glucose level is not well known. They may do other damage, and may also contribute to impaired judgment and risk-taking behaviors such as unprotected intercourse.

Alcohol

Drinking alcohol without precautions can lead to hypoglycemia, because alcohol interferes with the liver's natural ability to make sugar and add it to the bloodstream. Furthermore, under the influence of alcohol, a teen may miss the early warning symptoms of hypoglycemia and progress quickly to a severe episode. This may not be recognized by others who have also been drinking, or who, smelling alcohol on the teen's breath, presume he or she has "passed out" from being drunk.

As a general rule, it's better to educate teens with diabetes about alcohol use than to forbid it. They should understand that drinking in moderation is acceptable once they reach the legal drinking age, but that excessive alcohol use will put them at risk. They should always wear or carry identification stating that they have diabetes, in case of a hypoglycemic event. They should also learn to eat when they drink, to avoid hypoglycemia.

Contraception

Teens with diabetes sometimes wonder if they will be able to have children. We know that diabetes does not alter the fertility of young men, nor does it interfere with a young woman's ability to become pregnant. However, in order to best ensure a full-term healthy baby, the young woman with diabetes must plan her pregnancy so that she maintains excellent control both prior to conception and throughout the pregnancy.

All sexually active girls require contraception to prevent unplanned pregnancies. Generally speaking, the same options are available to women with diabetes as to those without.

Women who choose oral contraception, as well as sexually active young men, should use a condom to reduce the risk of sexually transmitted diseases. Sexually active teens should consider intercourse an extra activity that uses up energy, requiring a carbohydrate snack afterward.

Teens with diabetes should be provided with information about sexuality, contraception and pregnancy well in advance of needing it. These discussions should take place with members of the diabetes team, and should be confidential.

Eating Disorders

Eating disorders are common among teenage and young adult women, and are much less common among males in the same age group. Researchers believe they stem from an obsession about gaining control in a life they perceive to be out of control. There are many possible causes of this obsession, depending on the individual's experience. People with *anorexia nervosa* try to regain control by denying themselves food; people with *bulimia nervosa* try to regain control by excessive overeating (binging), then purging by self-induced vomiting or with the aid of laxatives. These definitions aren't cut and dried—people with one disorder sometimes exhibit characteristics of the other. In the long term, anorexia can lead to severe weight loss and can be fatal. The constant binging and purging of bulimia can result in severe stomach ulcers and can also be fatal.

In teenage and young adult women with Type 1 diabetes, disturbances in eating attitudes and behavior are common and persistent. Full-blown eating disorders are less common, but even milder disturbances can play havoc with blood glucose control.

Some diabetes-related factors may increase the likelihood of an eating disturbance. At the time of diagnosis there has often been weight loss. With insulin therapy this weight is quickly regained. In the vulnerable girl this may trigger dissatisfaction with her body and the desire to be thinner again. Also, meal planning is an integral part of diabetes treatment. Such planning implies a degree of dietary restraint, another trigger to disordered eating. Finally, some girls discover that by skipping or reducing their insulin dose, they can lose sugar in their urine and keep themselves underweight. Although this may be an effective way to control weight, it invariably leads to poor diabetes control and, in the long run, earlier onset of diabetes-related complications.

Warnings Signs of an Eating Disorder

Eating disorders in people with Type 1 diabetes can lead to wild, unexplained fluctuations in blood glucose levels, often outside the safe range. Frequent low glucose reactions (insulin reactions) or high glucose reactions (excessive thirst and urination, perhaps leading to urinary ketones) may be a sign that an eating disorder is complicating diabetes management. Eating disorders can also be marked by:

- a preoccupation with food and weight, beyond what is required in diabetes management
- a stated desire to lose weight beyond what seems appropriate
- requests for dietary change with low-calorie, low-fat, vegetarian or other diets to lose weight
- binge-eating episodes
- insulin manipulation

What You Can Do to Help

If you know someone with an eating disorder, there are several things you can do to help.

- Express your concern for the person's health, while respecting the need for privacy. Eating disorders are usually a symptom of a greater psychological problem, and the fact that you are there to help will be appreciated.

- Avoid power struggles around food. Forcing someone with an eating disorder to eat will probably make things worse.
- Examine your own attitudes around food and weight. Are you furthering the idea that "thin is in"?
- Talk about more flexible meal plans with your diabetes dietitian. Perhaps the current meal plan is too restrictive, reinforcing the idea that the person with diabetes is different and deprived.
- Avoid commenting on weight, either positively or negatively, as it only serves to emphasize the importance of appearance.
- Express your concern to your diabetes health care team and get support for the person.

Driving

Driving a car requires accurate judgment and a keen sense of responsibility. Young people with diabetes have an additional responsibility to ensure that their blood sugar is right before they get behind the wheel of a car. Low blood sugar can impair judgment, increasing the risk of an accident. Parents should be certain that teens show responsible self-management before permitting them to apply for a driver's license or lending them the family vehicle. Getting a regular driver's license is not generally a problem, as long as blood sugar control is reasonable and there have been no severe episodes of hypoglycemia in the previous year.

Employment

There are countless examples of people with diabetes who have excelled in a broad range of careers—doctors, lawyers, nurses, politicians, professional athletes, psychologists, accountants, researchers, teachers and engineers, to mention a few. In general, parents and educators find that young people can be coached and counseled to pursue the career that interests them or for which they have an aptitude. However, it is also important to be aware of current limitations. Two questions are often asked of the diabetes team: "Are there jobs that are not available to people with diabetes?" and "Do some employers discriminate against people with diabetes?" The answer to both questions is yes.

A number of organizations have a blanket rule that prevents employment of people with diabetes. Such employment includes jobs that require operation of a commercial vehicle such as a truck or an aircraft, and jobs in some military or police departments. These rules are based on the risk of hypoglycemia while on the job. Before applying for a particular educational or employment opportunity, teens with diabetes should inquire as to their employability in these areas.

Employer discrimination has been documented over many years. There is often a misconception that people with diabetes will attend their jobs less frequently and perform less effectively than their peers. Young job-seekers with diabetes should stress their personal qualifications, abilities and ambitions to potential employers. They should not withhold information about their diabetes, but rather stress the fact that they can perform as well as others. If they believe they are being treated unfairly, they should seek advice through their advocacy group, such as the Canadian or American Diabetes Association.

Jackie is 14 and has had diabetes since the age of seven. She's proud of the fact that she manages her diabetes independently. She checks her blood sugar three or four times a day, and takes her insulin three times a day. Already she participates in decisions about insulin dose adjustment. Her hemoglobin A_{1c} checks have been consistently in the 7s, indicating excellent blood sugar control. She's happy and involved in school and extracurricular activities.

At a recent clinic visit, the doctor discovered that, on one of the few occasions when Jackie's blood sugar checks were high, she recorded a lower result. When this was pointed out to Jackie she became very tearful. With a little prompting she was able to tell her diabetes nurse that she felt sad and upset because she was looking forward to a youth group trip to Ottawa, and her parents had agreed that she could go if she maintained "good" diabetes control; she believed that they wouldn't let her go if they saw the high blood sugar results. Jackie asked her nurse to help her explain the doctor's discovery and her feelings and concerns to her mother, who was in the waiting room.

Jackie's mom listened to the explanation, and tears welled up in her eyes. She put her arm around her daughter, saying, "Jackie, that's not what your father and I meant by 'good' control. We should have been clearer about what we expected." In fact, all her parents meant was that she should put in a strong effort. Everyone has occasional highs and lows, sometimes for no apparent reason, and Jackie's parents didn't mean to suggest that they expected perfection. The misunderstanding opened up the opportunity for Jackie and her parents to clarify and renegotiate their goals.

Helpful Hints for All Ages

- *Get everyone in the family involved.* Diabetes care is a partnership between the child and the entire family. Mothers often shoulder a major share of the responsibility, but fathers need to be part of this as well. Talk about your feelings in an open manner. On the other hand, try not to let diabetes become the focus of every family meal or discussion. Also, recruit the support of others—grandparents, camp counselors, schoolteachers, sports coaches. The more they know about your child, the more comfortable you'll feel when they're in charge.

- *Set realistic blood sugar targets.* Expecting every blood sugar to be, say, 8 mmol/L (144 mg/dL) is unrealistic. In fact, it's impossible! Good diabetes control means balancing all the aspects of your life and lifestyle, not just focusing on blood sugar results.
- *Make good use of your diabetes team.* Don't be afraid to ask questions. And ask more questions if the answers don't seem to fit. (See more about getting the most out of your diabetes team in Chapter Ten.)
- *Take credit for trying, and don't feel bad about mistakes— they're bound to happen.* Diabetes is a complex and often frustrating condition. Doing the same thing two days in a row does not always lead to the same results.
- *Experiment a little and see what works for you and your child.* What you learn in your diabetes education and clinic sessions provides you with an excellent foundation. You've become a mini-expert in diabetes. But you haven't been given every answer to every question. Also, some things work better for some people. Use your knowledge to experiment a little. For example, taking less of the appropriate insulin before a sports game may work better in your family than eating a large amount of extra food.
- *Be realistic in your expectations of what responsibility your child will take for the diabetes.* Don't expect too much too soon. On the other hand, try not to be overbearing and overprotective.

- *Be careful to praise good performance.* It's very easy to focus on the negatives. "You're late for your blood sugar check!" "Did you take your insulin yet?" It's also easy to overlook the positives. Try not to. Praise every little advance, and look for opportunities for ongoing education when things are a little off track.
- *Make some time for yourself and your spouse or significant other.* Sometimes the diabetes seems to take up every minute of every day, and you feel as if you have no time for the things you have always loved to do—read a book, take a walk, go to a movie. Your child needs you to be in as good shape as he or she is. Have fun for yourself and also for your child.

Q&A

It takes half an hour of bargaining to get my three-year-old to cooperate during injection time. How can I make this go more smoothly?

It's not unusual for children of all ages to go through periods when they cry, squirm and use all kinds of delaying tactics to avoid insulin injections and finger pricks. Sometimes it's because the needle hurts. More often they are angry about being held still or having their play interrupted. Remember how hard it is just to wipe a toddler's nose! They may also be reacting to the fear and anxiety they sense in you. Here are some helpful hints for making injection time go more smoothly:

- Try to take a "matter of fact" approach to the insulin injections and finger pricks.
- Be quick, calm and reassuring when you carry out these routines.
- Reduce your child's anxious time by getting the dose and/or equipment ready before you involve the child.

- If possible, go where the child is playing to cause less disruption.
- Your child's crying, protests and other delaying tactics are normal. Remember that, each time you give insulin or do a finger prick, you are helping your child stay healthy.
- Gently hold or restrain your child if he or she struggles.
- Get the needle or finger prick over with quickly. Delaying it only prolongs the agony for everyone.
- Give your child a big hug and kiss after you give the needle, even if he or she didn't cooperate.
- Praise your child for any sign of cooperation.

Can diabetes complicate menstruation?
No, but the hormonal increase during menstruation can cause blood sugar levels to rise. Some women require more insulin during their periods. This is checked by observing the blood sugar pattern during the menstrual cycle.

Can I sleep in on weekends?
Although your diabetes team stresses consistency in the timing of meals and snacks, with a little extra effort and caution you can make the adjustments needed to sleep in safely. For example, if you're going to bed at midnight on Saturday night and you want to sleep in until 10 a.m. Sunday, try this: instead of taking your evening NPH insulin at 10 p.m., take it at midnight, together with a blood sugar check and a little extra snack. (If you're on two injections a day, it's advisable to split the evening one: take the fast-acting insulin before supper, and take the intermediate-acting at bedtime, along with an added small snack and a blood sugar check.) This will ensure that you don't go low during those extra sleep hours.

Can someone with diabetes learn to fly a plane?
People with diabetes have recently challenged the FAA in the United States, and Transport Canada, to reverse a blanket policy banning anyone with diabetes from flying a plane. Now, recreational pilots with diabetes are determined fit for flying based on their individual records of blood glucose control.

I get tired of always being the "bad guy," always saying no when my 12-year-old asks for a treat other than at a meal or snack time—any suggestions?
Some parents handle this situation by reversing the question: "Well, what do you think? Do you think you can have that treat and still keep your blood sugar balanced?" Most often, the child makes a sensible choice. Sometimes the question leads to creative problem-solving.

My nine-year-old learned to give his own insulin injection at camp last summer and continued to do it regularly for the month after camp. But now he's lost interest and doesn't want to do it anymore. Should we insist that he carry on?
No. It's appropriate for you to take most of the responsibility for injections right now. He'll do it again when he's motivated. If he wants to go on a sleepover he'll have to show you, a little while in advance, that he can safely manage this task.

Another tactic is to pull out a calendar and plan, together, a few days when he's going to give his shot with your supervision. This will maintain his confidence level.

My six-year-old son has been forgetting to eat his morning snack at school. He's been arriving home quite low at lunch some days. What should I do?
In general, six-year-olds have no concept of time—and playing

in the schoolyard often takes precedence over eating a snack. It's unlikely your son is going to remember to take that snack on his own, and it's reasonable to expect your son's teacher to remind him when it's time. If the snack is interfering with play, consider something fast and easy to eat: for example, a few raisins instead of an apple. Or, if necessary, ask the teacher to give him the snack in class just prior to the recess break.

I have a hard time getting my teen to do a blood sugar check. I know from attending a parents' group meeting that other parents have the same problem. It just takes a few minutes out of their day. Why is it such a problem getting these important checks done?

There are a lot of reasons why teens hate checking their blood sugar levels:

- It's inconvenient and time-consuming—to a teen, losing a few minutes of sleep or party time means a lot.
- Each check is a reminder that they have diabetes and they are not the same as their peers.
- They feel accountable for each blood sugar result—parents frequently demand explanations for high or low readings.
- The results may make them feel guilty—they may know why they're high but be unwilling to do anything about it. It feels better not to check.
- They don't understand the purpose of checking—they don't know how to use the results.
- They feel discouraged by the results, which don't reflect their efforts to manage their diabetes.

It's worthwhile having a discussion with your teen in an attempt to discover what the issues are in his or her particular case.

Putting Complications in Perspective

To 22-year-old Jason, those early days of learning about diabetes are like a long-ago nightmare. They started a little more than ten years ago, when all he could think of was not missing a hockey game. Now he's thinking about his future. He's almost finished university. He's in love with a girl he met in second year. Will he get a job? Will he get married? Intermingled with thoughts of career and personal relationships are anxieties about his diabetes in the next stage of his life. Will the disease interfere with his long-term plans? If so, what can he do to lessen the risk? His parents have been concerned about these things for years!

After the discovery of insulin, diabetes was no longer immediately life-threatening. Doctors expected that all the problems of the disease would disappear too. Unfortunately this was not the case, and a new set of diabetes-related complications soon began to emerge. Over the last several decades, researchers have learned a great deal about these complications—their symptoms, causes and treatment—and how to slow their progression. Perhaps most important, researchers are now devising ways to prevent complications altogether. *The best way to prevent complications from diabetes is to maintain the best blood glucose control possible.* This is hard work and, because complications are very rare in young people, the threat rarely motivates them. Most young people seldom think about their health 20 years down the road, and children with diabetes are no exception. That's where parents, family members and health care professionals come in—to provide the foresight and support to help them stay on track toward a healthy future.

The list of potential complications is long and can be quite depressing. But remember, these problems don't affect everyone with diabetes. We also know much more now about how to reduce the risk than even ten years ago.

What Are the Complications of Diabetes?

The physical complications fall into two groups: microvascular (involving small blood vessels) and macrovascular (involving large blood vessels).

Microvascular complications include:
- retinopathy, or eye damage
- nephropathy, or kidney damage
- neuropathy, or nerve damage

Macrovascular complications include:
- cardiovascular disease, or risk of heart attack
- cerebrovascular disease, or risk of stroke
- peripheral vascular disease, or poor circulation to the limbs, which may cause foot problems

While microvascular complications occur only in people with diabetes, macrovascular complications represent an *increased* risk of conditions that also occur in the general population.

These complications are virtually unheard of in young children and uncommon during the teenage years. However, diabetes probably starts to have its effect from the time of onset. The impact may be minimal before puberty, but early changes seem to accelerate during adolescence, so maintaining a good blood sugar balance right from the time of diagnosis will contribute to overall long-term health.

Risk Factors for the Development of Diabetes-related Complications:

- *Duration of diabetes:* Even the very earliest stages of these complications are rare in those who have had the disease for less than five years, and before the onset of puberty. After that, the longer the duration of the diabetes, the more likely it is that complications will arise.

- *Inadequate blood glucose control:* The Diabetes Control and Complications Trial showed a close relationship between both the onset and the progression of diabetes-related complications, and the degree of long-term blood sugar control. This trial demonstrated clearly that *control counts*. Independent of any other risk factors, excellent blood glucose control decreases the development of complications. However, that doesn't mean that someone with poor control is 100 percent guaranteed to have complications, nor does it mean that someone with excellent control is guaranteed not to have them.

- *Smoking:* Many studies show that smokers with diabetes are at much greater risk of developing complications, and having those complications worsen rapidly, than non-smokers. Giving up smoking decreases the risk considerably.

- *High blood pressure:* People with diabetes who develop high blood pressure (hypertension) are at high risk of complications because of increased pressure on the kidneys, heart and blood vessels. Lowering the blood pressure with aggressive medical treatment reduces this risk. Regular blood pressure checks are an essential part of diabetes care.

- *High blood fats (lipids—cholesterol and triglycerides):* People with poor blood glucose control develop high blood fat levels (*hyperlipidemia*). There are also people who are born with a tendency to develop high blood fat levels. In both cases, these high levels contribute to the risk of complications. Screening for high blood fats is another important part of diabetes care.

Blood glucose and complications— what's the connection?

Although we know that persistently high blood glucose levels are associated with an increased risk of complications, the connection between the two is still the subject of intense research. It's likely that a number of different mechanisms are involved. For example, glucose sticks to many proteins (as it sticks to hemoglobin, leading to the formation of HbA$_{1c}$). Over a long period the attachment of the glucose may change the way some proteins function, and damage the surrounding tissues. This suggestion is called the *glucotoxicity theory.*

High blood sugar levels also affect the metabolism of many tissues, by altering the rate at which certain molecules are produced or removed. This may lead to a decreased level of molecules that are essential to the way the tissue functions, or the level may be increased enough to damage tissues. Among the tissues affected this way are the nerves and the lens of the eye.

When poor blood glucose control leads to high levels of fat in the blood, that fat may be deposited in the arteries, causing arteriosclerosis (hardening of the arteries)—a major risk factor for macrovascular diseases such as heart attack and stroke. People with diabetes are more likely to develop high blood pressure, which increases the risk of arteriosclerosis and is in itself a risk factor for macrovascular disease.

• *Obesity:* People who are markedly overweight are at increased risk for macrovascular complications. Weight control may be a difficult challenge for teens and adults, especially girls.

Screening for Complications in Youth

It is very unusual for children under the age of puberty, or those with diabetes for less than three to five years, to show evidence of long-term complications. Even in teens who have had diabetes for five or ten years, advanced complications are extremely unusual. Nevertheless, once puberty has started and the disease has been present for three to five years, screening for complications and risk factors should begin. If no problems are found, that's reassuring. If the early stages of complications are detected, that allows intervention to prevent them from developing, or at least to slow their progression.

Here are some blood and urine tests and examinations that your health care team will recommend on a regular basis. More frequent testing will likely be advised if any abnormalities are discovered.

Test/Examination	Frequency
Blood pressure	every 3–6 months
HbA_{1c} (to assess metabolic control)	every 3–4 months
Laboratory blood sugar against your own meter (to check your meter's accuracy)	every 3–6 months

Thyroid function (thyroid stimulating hormone—to detect overfunctioning or underfunctioning of the thyroid)	annually
Blood fats (cholesterol and triglycerides)	3–6 months after diagnosis and, if normal, once again after puberty
Overnight or 24-hour urine collection for microalbuminuria, or albumin: creatinine ratio in a random urine sample (to detect early diabetic nephropathy)	annually after onset of puberty and 3–5 years of diabetes
Eye checkup with ophthalmologist (to detect early diabetic retinopathy)	annually after onset of puberty and 5 years of diabetes
Dental checkups	every 6 months

Diabetic Retinopathy

Diabetic retinopathy is damage to the *retina*, the light-sensitive lining at the back of the eyeball. The condition starts quietly and slowly, with changes seen only on careful examination of the eye by an experienced ophthalmologist. In its early and even late stages, retinopathy does not usually interfere with vision. Once vision impairment begins, it suggests that the retinopathy is far advanced.

The earliest changes are called *background (non-proliferative) retinopathy*, and consist of little swellings of the blood vessels, called *microaneurysms*, which may start to leak or burst causing exudates (leaking) and hemorrhages (bleeding). Vision is only compromised if the bleeding affects the *macula* (the part of the eye that focuses on the object of vision), or if that area swells (*macular edema*). Almost everyone with Type 1 diabetes will develop background retinopathy after having the disease for 15 to 20 years.

Anatomy of the eye

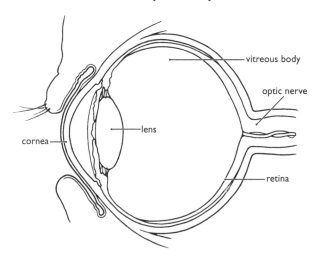

This early stage of retinopathy may progress to *proliferative retinopathy*, where the eye begins to make new blood vessels to provide better blood flow. These new vessels are fragile and may cause bleeding and scarring in the fluid chamber (vitreous body) in front of the retina. This bleeding is called *vitreous hemorrhage*, and the scarring can cause detachment of the retina. Proliferative retinopathy and its consequences are a major cause of partial or complete loss of sight. In developed countries, diabetic retinopathy is the most common cause of acquired blindness in adults. However, this does not mean that most people with diabetes will lose their vision.

Researchers have made great strides in repairing vision and reducing the risk of blindness in people with diabetes. Photocoagulation is a laser therapy technique that prevents blindness by destroying abnormal blood vessels, repairing leaking ones and stopping new ones from forming. This should reduce the risk of blindness by more than 75–80 percent. Occasionally, if the retina has bled too much or has become detached, surgery may be required.

Cataracts

A cataract is a thickening in the lens of the eye. The sugar alcohol *sorbitol*, a byproduct of high blood sugar, is believed to be the cause. Cataracts cause persistent blurring of vision. They are very rarely found in young people with Type 1 diabetes, but can develop at any time.

Cataracts can be surgically removed, and the remaining visual impairment corrected with glasses or contact lenses.

Nephropathy

The two kidneys are the body's filtering system. As blood flows through the blood vessels into the kidneys, toxins and waste are removed and transported out of the kidneys, and out of the body, in the urine. The relationship between diabetes and kidney disease is complex. Kidneys may enlarge and become overworked, in a condition called *diabetic nephropathy*.

Not all people with Type 1 diabetes develop nephropathy. It is more likely to occur after puberty, in about one in three people who have had Type 1 diabetes for 15 years or longer. Poor blood glucose control, high blood pressure and smoking (or chewing) tobacco also increase the risk of kidney failure.

Normal retina

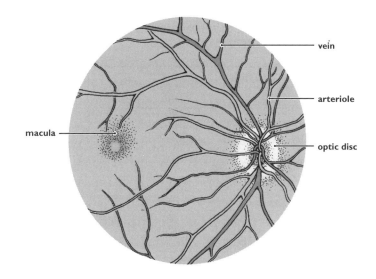

Retinopathy

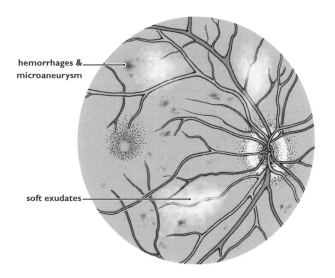

Nephropathy, like retinopathy, develops slowly and quietly, with no symptoms or signs until serious kidney damage has occurred. Symptoms and signs may include:

- higher blood pressure than usual
- puffy ankles due to water retention (*edema*)
- excessive protein in the urine (*proteinuria*)
- excessive waste levels in the blood (*high concentration of creatinine and urea*)

Diabetic nephropathy can be detected at a very early stage, before it causes symptoms. This early phase, called *incipient nephropathy*, is marked by the presence of very small amounts of the protein albumin in the urine. This is called *microalbuminuria* and is detected in a 24-hour or overnight urine specimen. If nephropathy progresses, the amount of protein in the urine will steadily increase to the stage of *overt proteinuria*. Now protein can be detected by means of a routine protein dipstick in the urine.

Recent research has demonstrated that the onset of diabetic nephropathy can be prevented, or its progression can be significantly slowed, by achieving and maintaining excellent blood glucose control. Further progression can also be prevented or slowed with specific medications (called *angiotensin converting enzyme* or *ACE inhibitors*).

If nephropathy remains untreated, it will progress to chronic renal (kidney) failure and eventually to end-stage renal failure, which requires dialysis or transplantation if the person is to survive.

Advanced nephropathy is associated with a significant increased risk of macrovascular complications and early death due to diabetes.

Neuropathy

High blood sugars over the long term can also affect the nerves in many areas of the body. Some slowing of the electrical impulses which travel along the nerves is common in people with diabetes. However, some people go on to develop symptoms and signs of more severe neuropathy. This is extremely rare in children or teens.

Neuropathy commonly affects the nerves to the arms and the legs, and is characterized by:

• tingling in the fingers and toes, extending toward the body
• numbness (loss of feeling) in these areas
• painful burning or freezing sensations, particularly in the feet
• cramping or weakness
• inability to detect hot and cold temperatures

Symptoms of neuropathy can come and go, and are influenced by the level of blood sugar control. Certain prescription medications (such as the antidepressant imipramine, or the anticonvulsants mexiletine or clonazepam) may alleviate the pain.

Autonomic neuropathy, which is distinctly unusual in childhood or adolescence, affects the nerves to internal organs, such as the gastrointestinal system or bladder. When the gastrointestinal system is affected, there may be problems with the stomach (including vomiting and difficulty moving the food into the intestines, along with bloating) or with the intestines (including constipation or, more commonly, diarrhea). Therapy is difficult, but may include smaller meal sizes and medications to improve intestinal action.

Nerve damage affecting the bladder can lead to urine retention or loss of bladder control. In some cases, men experience sexual dysfunction or impotence. These problems can be improved significantly with better blood glucose control and, if needed, medication.

Foot Problems

The risk of foot problems in children and adolescents with diabetes is negligible. As people with diabetes get older, they are more susceptible to infections and slow healing, due to poor circulation and the effects of neuropathy. A person with neuropathy can get a cut on the sole of the foot, or a blister from an ill-fitting shoe, and not even know it. This is especially likely to happen if the injury is the first indicator of neuropathy, and the feet are not being examined each day. If the cut remains unnoticed, it can quickly become infected and, in the worst case, lead to gangrene (tissue death). The only recourse then is to amputate the dead tissue.

Although children don't usually experience foot infections, poor healing or gangrene, it's wise for them to develop good foot care habits so that problems can be avoided as they get older. From an early age, they should be taught how to take good care of their feet, just as they learn how to take good care of their hair, teeth and other parts of their body. Good foot care means keeping the feet clean and dry—just as anyone would—wearing proper-fitting shoes, cutting toenails straight across rather than rounding them, avoiding ingrown toenails and getting into the habit of examining the feet for cuts and blisters on a regular basis.

Macrovascular Complications

As people age, so do their large blood vessels. The term for this aging process is *arteriosclerosis* (often called "hardening of the arteries"). People with Type 1 diabetes are susceptible to early aging of their large blood vessels, as are people who

---

A good health reminder

The Diabetes Control and Complications Trial proved that the risk of developing macrovascular complications can be significantly reduced with careful attention to blood glucose levels. Children can also decrease their risk of complications in adulthood by adopting healthy habits now:

- Eat a healthy diet to maintain normal blood fats and body weight.
- Don't smoke. Every day the list of complications of cigarette smoke gets longer. The effects of smoking are compounded in people with diabetes.
- Keep your blood pressure down. If the body has to work harder than it should to pump blood, the blood vessels and kidneys start to feel the effects. Eye problems may also be aggravated by high blood pressure. You can lower blood pressure by exercising, eating properly (with less salt) and maintaining a healthy weight.
- Get regular exercise, but work it into your plan.

---

smoke, are obese, have persistently high blood fats or have uncontrolled high blood pressure. Arteriosclerosis can lead to heart attacks or heart failure (cardiovascular disease), strokes (cerebrovascular disease) or foot problems (peripheral vascular disease). As in other complications of diabetes, the risk can be reduced by maintaining excellent blood glucose control, keeping blood pressure in check, exercising regularly, eating a healthy diet and not smoking.

Macrovascular complications are an ominous sign. Fortunately, they are almost unheard of in teens.

Q&A

Is it all right for my six-year-old daughter with diabetes to go barefoot at the beach?
If you think it is safe for anyone in your family to walk around with bare feet on the beach, then it should be safe for your daughter too. At her age, your daughter will have no more trouble healing than other members of the family.

Will our child have difficulty obtaining life insurance policies or any other types of insurance, such as mortgage, car or home insurance, because of the diabetes?

In the past, insurance companies either were unwilling to provide coverage or else demanded a significantly higher rate for life and other insurance policies for people with diabetes. More recently, with improved care and a better long-term outlook, most insurance companies have become increasingly willing to provide this coverage. It is important that people with diabetes, like anyone else in society, have appropriate insurance. Shop around for the best policies and prices available. Ask advice of your local diabetes association or support group, or others you know who have diabetes. Also, don't take no for an answer if your first attempts to get coverage are refused. Keep requesting coverage, and ask your doctor or other health professional to write a letter supporting your application.

Is my child more likely to need glasses because of the diabetes?

Children with diabetes are no more likely than their non-diabetic friends to need glasses for either near- or farsightedness. Diabetes does not cause permanent problems with vision unless retinopathy has become severe. This is exceptionally rare during childhood and adolescence. Sometimes, rapid changes in blood sugar can cause changes to the lens of the eye—swelling (if the sugar is very high) or contraction (if the sugar is very low). This can cause temporary blurring of vision. Balancing the blood sugar will invariably correct this. Nevertheless, a child who complains of difficulty seeing the chalkboard, or has to sit close to the television, should have an eye exam to see if glasses are required.

My teenage daughter has diabetes. So far her doctor has not recommended any special eye or kidney tests. Is this OK?
It may be that your doctor has not initiated these checks because your daughter has had diabetes for less than five years. Regular screening should start after the onset of puberty and should also be done for children who have had diabetes longer than five years. If your daughter has had diabetes for that long, don't hesitate to bring up your concerns with your doctor; ask for a referral to an ophthalmologist (eye specialist), and request a urine check for microalbuminuria.

My teenage son has diabetes and his doctor is recommending that he begin regular eye exams with an ophthalmologist instead of the optometrist I see. What is the difference between these two eye doctors?
For people with diabetes, the purpose of regular eye examinations is both to check visual acuity (how well they see) and to examine the interior of the eye for any signs of damage (retinopathy) which, left untreated, may interfere with vision. The follow-up and treatment of any retinopathy require the expertise of an ophthalmologist, a physician who specializes in the diagnosis and treatment (both medical and surgical) of eye disorders. An optometrist, who is not a physician, specializes in measuring the refractive power of the lens of the eye and fitting people with glasses or contact lenses. Like the ophthalmologist, the optometrist is expected to put drops in your son's eyes to dilate the pupils in order to do a thorough examination of the back of the eye, using special equipment. Should any retinopathy be detected, your son should be referred to an ophthalmologist, if he is not already seeing one.

Does having diabetes mean that my child is more likely to develop kidney or bladder infections?

Poorly controlled diabetes with very high sugar readings, especially in girls, may lead to an increased susceptibility to bladder or vaginal infections. Diabetic nephropathy (kidney damage) does not cause an increased risk of kidney or bladder infection.

Do oral contraceptives increase the risk of diabetes-related complications?
Research shows that women with diabetes who use the "pill" are not at any greater risk of complications than those who use other forms of contraception. The pills used today have much lower dosages of estrogen (the female hormone) than previously.

Is smoking really bad for people with diabetes?
Yes! There are stacks of research to show that people with diabetes who choose to smoke are at greater risk for developing both microvascular and macrovascular complications. Also, they are likely to take more time off work or school when they have minor illnesses such as a cold or flu.

I have heard that impotence is a complication of diabetes in men. Is this true?
Some men do experience impotence as a complication of diabetes. This may be the result of nerve damage and circulation problems associated with long-standing diabetes and inadequate blood sugar control. Careful attention to diabetes self-management and blood glucose control is the best way to stay healthy and prevent impotence.

TEN

Setting the Stage for a Healthy Future

On his sixteenth birthday, Paul reached more than one milestone. Soon he would be driving a car, but it was also his tenth year of living with diabetes. Unfortunately, getting Paul to keep diabetes clinic appointments has become increasingly difficult. Either they conflict with an important game or exam, or he complains that, since he feels fine and his blood sugar levels are fine, why should he have to go to the clinic? It's a good thing that Paul's blood sugar levels are so stable. But even when things are going well, there are reasons to stay in touch with the diabetes team. Paul is missing out on the opportunity to learn about changes in diabetes care. For instance, an athlete like Paul would probably benefit from a four-shot-a-day insulin routine, but Paul is behind the times. Also, as Paul gets older he needs to become aware of prevention and screening of complications that may affect him in adulthood. In order to re-establish a baseline and to detect possible changes in eye, kidney or nerve function, Paul has to see his diabetes team regularly.

As soon as the diagnosis of Type 1 diabetes is made, insulin therapy begins and parents and child start an education program to take them through the basics of diabetes management. Once early stabilization and initial education are complete, the major challenge is to maintain health and well-being, both short-term and long-term. This requires regular visits and consultation with the diabetes team, and education updates, to prepare the family for new periods in growth and psychosocial development. The continuing focus on health maintenance and health promotion helps motivate and encourage persistent and careful attention to diabetes management. Most of the time, families are able to avoid, or at least deal with, crises before they get out of hand. There are planned educational and support sessions to smooth the transition from one stage of development to the next. In particular, the regular follow-up helps pave the way for the teen to transfer to an adult care diabetes team toward the end of adolescence.

Health Care Follow-up

Ongoing follow-up is essential. Clinical Practice Guidelines published by both the Canadian and American Diabetes Association suggest a minimum of three or four visits per year (every three or four months), and more in the first year of diabetes and for those on an intensive management regimen.

Reasons for regular follow-up include:
- assessment of
  - health in general and diabetes in particular
  - growth and development
  - attitudes and behaviors, including school attendance
  - lifestyle issues, e.g. current activities—sleeping in, smoking, alcohol use

- current and anticipated challenges in living with and coping with diabetes management
- updating and/or clarifying goals and expectations
- anticipatory guidance and joint problem-solving with various members of the team
- support and reassurance
- ongoing education—for parents, children and teens to learn new skills, concepts and management measures, and to review important principles and practices
- ensuring surveillance for diabetes-related complications, when appropriate
- finding out what is new in research
- having the opportunity to participate in relevant research

The Clinic Visit
Clinic visits are a time to take stock of how well the diabetes is being controlled, how it impacts on the child's and family's lifestyle and how their lifestyle is affecting the diabetes. Visits focus on three areas:
- *diabetes-specific issues* such as:
    - insulin requirements (frequency, injection sites, timing of injections, types of insulin, dosages)
    - meal planning (including eating attitudes and behavior, particularly in adolescents)
    - results of self-monitoring of blood glucose levels
    - symptoms, frequency and treatment of hypoglycemia and hyperglycemia
    - physical and other activities that affect blood glucose control
    - sick days
- *growth and physical development*, including progression of puberty

- *psychosocial adjustment*, including family stress, school attendance and performance, behavioral issues and, in the teen, issues such as smoking, alcohol and drug usage, sexuality and sexual exploration, career planning and, eventually, transition to adult care

The physical checkup generally includes height and weight measurements to ensure that the child is growing well. The doctor or nurse will also measure blood pressure, feel the thyroid gland (in the neck) and the liver for any enlargement, look at the back of the eye with an ophthalmoscope and inspect insulin injection sites for bumps and lumps.

In addition to letting the diabetes team monitor physical changes, the regular visits also afford parents and child an opportunity to learn more about diabetes, and become more confident in their ability to make their own routine adjustments. The diabetes team can also help identify any potential psychosocial issues that may affect diabetes management, or vice versa, and begin to deal with them immediately and appropriately.

Since the needs of children with diabetes change as they age, it helps if children and their families can continue to meet the members of their core diabetes team for refresher courses. Many centers offer group meetings where parents can meet other parents and ask questions of experts, while children meet other children with diabetes in a friendly environment. However, some individual family counseling is also advisable because it nurtures the relationship between the team and the growing child or teen. While these sessions are imperative for children who are having a hard time achieving blood glucose targets, they are also a valuable support for those with excellent or good control.

Thyroid disease and diabetes

About one in four or five people with Type I diabetes will develop alterations in the function of the thyroid gland. While this is associated with diabetes, it is not a complication of long-standing or poorly controlled diabetes. The thyroid is found in the lower part of the front of the neck, and is responsible for production of the thyroid hormones (thyroxine or T4 and tri-iodothyronine or T3), which are important regulators of growth and metabolism.

The thyroid may be the target of an autoimmune response similar to the one that affects the beta cells in the pancreas and causes diabetes. This thyroid damage is known as Hashimoto's thyroiditis, and may cause underactivity of the thyroid gland *(hypothyroidism)*. If the thyroid starts to become underactive, the body's metabolism slows. This may reveal itself in slower growth, weight gain, tiredness or sluggishness, dry skin and hair, constipation and, in women, menstrual irregularities.

Regular checks of thyroid function allow detection of underactivity before symptoms become evident. Checks involve measuring the level of the hormone TSH, or *thyroid stimulating hormone*, made in the pituitary gland, in the brain. As the thyroid gland starts to fail, the pituitary gland makes more TSH in an attempt to bolster thyroid function. An elevated TSH level is therefore the best indicator of impending thyroid failure. If thyroid underactivity is detected, it can be treated with *levo-thyroxine*, a synthetic form of thyroid hormone, in the form of a small pill.

In rare instances the thyroid gland becomes overactive. Symptoms of hyperthyroidism (Graves' disease) may include weight loss with increased appetite, mood swings, shakiness and sweating, diarrhea and prominence of the eyes. This can be treated with thyroid-suppressing medications.

The Role of the Family Doctor

The relationship with the diabetes health care team cannot and should not replace the role of the family doctor or pediatrician in attending to the child's general health. Routine immunization, managing infections and annual physicals should continue outside the diabetes team. Good communication is essential. Parents and diabetes specialists should keep the family doctor informed about the child's diabetes management plan. Likewise, the family doctor will communicate any concerns to the rest of the diabetes team.

Getting the Most Out of the Visit with Your Health Care Team
Over the years the family dealing with diabetes will become quite familiar with the health care system. Some people take a while to become comfortable working with health care professionals, but remember that the diabetes team is there for the family. Here are some tips on how to get the most from your health care team.

Before the visit
- write out questions and concerns so you won't forget things
- write down any recent symptoms
- keep self-monitoring records current
- know and follow the standards of care
- know what the previous HbA$_{1c}$ was
- rehearse the main points you want to cover

During the visit
- remember to bring the blood glucose record book and the glucose meter
- request time to ask questions
- write down the answers
- repeat answers back to the health care provider for clarity
- make a specific plan of action for any changes to the diabetes routine
- make an appointment for the next visit
- ask if thyroid and blood fat tests should be done. If the child is over 15 years of age and has had diabetes for three to five years, ask if it is time to begin screening for eye and kidney changes

After the visit
- list the recommendations given
- decide to implement them
- tell the rest of the family
- encourage the child to keep a diary to help keep track of the routine
- phone to get the HbA_{1c} result from the previous visit as soon as it is available
- phone to get results from any other screening tests

Moving from Pediatric to Adult Health Care

Although children with diabetes have special needs and benefit from care given by health care providers experienced in childhood diabetes, there comes a time when the teenager needs to link up with a team experienced in the care of adults.

This transition can be quite emotional and stressful for all. Moving on to a new health care setting is like graduating from high school to college. Over a short period of time, the teenager shifts from being the biggest, oldest and wisest person to being a young, inexperienced rookie in a larger and different environment. Some find the experience exciting, while others prefer the security of the old setting. Expectations for self-management and control differ between pediatric and adult care. In the adult system, young adults are often seen as taking complete responsibility for themselves.

As teens enter the adult system, many are surprised by the demands placed on them. If they are not already doing so, they may be expected to practice intensive management of their diabetes, aiming for tighter blood sugar control through more frequent injections and glucose monitoring. There will be changes in meal plans, as they are no longer growing. Some find they are not as physically active as they used to be, and have to compensate for that with a more structured exercise regimen. As their risk of complications increases with age, they may have to monitor blood pressure and see an eye doctor more frequently. Routine foot care will be emphasized, to prevent infections and identify signs of nerve damage. These demands can be overwhelming and the newly graduated teenager can feel incapable of meeting them. Some young adults are tempted to drop out of care altogether. The support of family and friends throughout the transition phase is vital to ensure that the young adult continues with the care needed to manage his or her diabetes.

Ideally, the change to adult care should come when the teenager is confident and responsible enough to move forward. Unfortunately, hospital or clinic policy usually dictates a transition between the ages of 16 and 20. Parents and teens should be aware of this well ahead of time in order to prepare.

Parents can help teens make a successful transfer by encouraging them to take an active part in their diabetes care throughout childhood and adolescence. When parents encourage their children to problem-solve and make choices about adjusting insulin doses, for example, they set the foundation for the self-management behaviors essential in adulthood. Teenagers also need private time with all members of the diabetes team, as this promotes independence and responsibility. Before being discharged from the pediatric center, teens should have the opportunity to explore various options for continuing their diabetes health care, and a referral should be made to the adult team. It is also helpful for a teen leaving the pediatric center to take part in either an individual or a group program that stresses the need for ongoing excellent blood glucose control, surveillance for complications and changing expectations.

Q&A

Our daughter has diabetes. Are there any special precautions we should take when we go on our summer holiday?
Your daughter's diabetes should not discourage you from traveling—even abroad. Unfortunately, you can't take a vacation from her diabetes. But careful planning will ensure a safe and enjoyable holiday. Here are some tips:

- Take enough insulin and other supplies to last for the entire trip, and some to spare. Keep the extra in a separate location from the main supply, in case one of your bags is lost or stolen.
- If you're boarding a plane, make sure all your supplies are in your carry-on baggage.
- Wherever you go, always carry some food, together with a good supply of fast-acting sugar to treat insulin reactions.
- Plan to monitor blood sugar at least three to four times a day—specifically, before meals and at bedtime. The routine will be different than it is at home, and you'll need to know how her blood sugar is affected so you can make safe adjustments.
- For active holidays, you may need to reduce your daughter's insulin. Speak with members of your diabetes team.
- Make sure your daughter wears some form of diabetes identification, such as a medical-alert bracelet.
- Be prepared for emergencies. Take the glucagon kit with you, so you can respond to severe low blood sugar if necessary. And take your sick-day guidelines and your ketone testing strips with you.
- Don't forget to take the phone numbers of key members of your diabetes team. They may also be able to provide you with the names of experts in your holiday location.

How do I deal with a time-zone change?
There is no magic formula to help you figure out how to adjust insulin for a time-zone change—every situation and individual is different. Know the time action of your insulins inside out, and gather all the information you can about your flight— time change and available food (you'll bring along extra, of course). Then sit down with your doctor or nurse to figure out a plan.

Is it hard to get travel insurance?
As with life and other forms of insurance, it can be more difficult for people with diabetes to obtain travel insurance. The diabetes association may offer travel insurance to members. Contact your nearest branch for more information.

My son wants to go on a ten-day camping trip into the wilderness. He will be out of contact with civilization for most of the time. Should I let him go?
This is a decision for you and your son to make. Before letting him go, you should feel comfortable that he and his friends understand the issues involved in being out in the wilderness. Your son should have demonstrated good judgment and a high level of responsibility in diabetes care, and should be committed to doing more, rather than less, blood sugar testing on the trip. You should make every effort to ensure that there is some method of communication with "civilization" if at all possible.

After my daughter "graduates" from the diabetes clinic at the hospital, isn't it OK for her to be seen by her family doctor only?
It's still important for your daughter to have access to all members of the diabetes health care team (doctor, nurse, dietit-

ian, social worker), even after she leaves the children's clinic. There are obstacles to negotiate at each age and stage of development, such as moving away to college or university, living on her own, changes in exercise or activity patterns, frequent trips away from home on business—the list goes on and on. These are best dealt with by health care professionals experienced in diabetes care. If your family doctor is one of these, then he or she may well meet your daughter's needs.

ELEVEN

The Future of Diabetes

Samantha is an inquisitive, freckle-faced girl who has had diabetes for six years. Now 13, she recently began giving her own injections. For the past three years she has been doing her blood glucose checks and she is comfortable taking some glucose tablets when she feels low at her skating lesson. At first Samantha didn't want to tell anybody, but within six months she gave her first "talk" to her grade two classmates about what it was like to have diabetes. Last year, she won an essay contest with her biography of Frederick Banting.

Samantha likes to surf the Web and often looks for innovations in diabetes. Perhaps one day she won't have to take insulin via injection any longer. At each clinic visit she has a long list of questions for her doctor about new research in diabetes.

Since the discovery of insulin, important advances in the understanding of the cause, course and complications of both Type 1 and Type 2 diabetes have continued to be made. But only some of these advances have led to significant changes in the lives of those with the disease. Others reflect a gain in our knowledge about diabetes. Media reports of "breakthroughs" often offer unrealistic hope to children with diabetes and their parents: hope that their lives are to be dramatically changed in the very near future. Reality is often different; advances in biomedical research usually take many years to proceed through the appropriate stages of testing, first in test-tubes, then in animals and finally in people. Another reality is that many advances in research, after some initially successful results, do not pan out. While these experiments may advance our understanding of disease in substantial ways, they may not offer new treatment approaches. So read the newspaper or watch the news with a critical eye, and get as much information as you can from health care professionals, diabetes journals and other sources before forming an opinion.

Some people with diabetes (as well as those with other conditions) are quite cynical, believing that the research and medical communities have the ability to cure their disease, but that there is too much profit to be made from not doing so. Nothing could be further from the truth. Both Type 1 and Type 2 diabetes pose a massive public health burden. It has been suggested that more than 10 percent of all health care expenditures are related in some way to diabetes. A cure is in everyone's best interests. However, a cure may be more elusive than the optimists or the media would have us believe.

Researching the Cause and Possible Cure

In Chapter One we talked about diabetes being an autoimmune disorder, caused when a genetic predisposition or susceptibility is triggered by an environmental stimulus. Over the past 20 years there have been enormous advances in our understanding of the genetic aspects of Type 1 diabetes, although pieces of the puzzle remain to be found.

The Genetic Link

There are a number of genes involved in making a person susceptible to Type 1 diabetes; the most important appears to lie in the HLA (histocompatibility locus antigen or "tissue typing") region of chromosome six. This region contains genes that control the body's immune responses—for example, how we deal with foreign materials such as viruses, bacteria and toxins. In those susceptible to diabetes, these genes appear to be somewhat impaired. Contained in this region of chromosome six are different genes that determine different levels of susceptibility, and some actually confer resistance to diabetes! Could this resistance be harnessed and turned into a gene therapy that could alter these impaired genes and protect against diabetes? This is an important research question, but the answer is still a long way off.

The Environmental Link

In the hunt for environmental triggers that may "wake up" a genetic predisposition to diabetes, there has been extensive research focusing on viruses, food products—such as exposure to cow's milk protein early in life—and environmental toxins. This research has not yielded consistent results, nor has it identified a single trigger for the development of diabetes. Researchers hope to identify a viral or other infectious agent responsible for causing the pancreatic damage, so they can work on developing a vaccine against it. This could conceivably prevent diabetes. Avoiding certain toxins could have a similar effect. There are studies in progress that test these hypotheses in both animals and humans.

Preventing the Immunological Response

Once the genes and environment align themselves in a way that starts the progression toward diabetes, a series of known events occur that are now quite well understood and are being studied in greater detail. The immune system and environmental abnormalities lead to an inflammatory response (*insulitis*) in the islet cells where insulin is made. Antibodies to some of the proteins in the islets appear in the blood. Detecting these antibodies allows us to determine who may be at high risk for developing diabetes.

Most of the studies have been and are being performed on close relatives (parents, children and siblings) of people with diabetes, because—as you'd expect in any disorder with a genetic link—the risk to family members is much higher than in the general population.

The problem is that diabetes in family members accounts for only 5 to 10 percent of all new cases of Type 1 diabetes. Studies in the general population have been much more difficult to perform, and may not be as useful for predictions as those in close relatives.

Studies in animals, such as certain breeds of mice and rats that spontaneously develop an autoimmune type of diabetes very similar to that seen in people, have shown that diabetes can be prevented by exposure to a number of medications that dampen the immunological response. These include some medications with serious side-effects, such as those used to prevent rejection of transplanted organs, as well as much safer agents, such as the vitamin derivative *nicotinamide* and the hormone insulin. Present studies in Canada, the United States and Europe are evaluating the possibility of preventing diabetes in high-risk groups by giving these medications.

Preventing the Progression of Diabetes

For those who already have diabetes, two different lines of

research are looking at ways to reverse the condition: immune interventions at diagnosis to stop further damage to the pancreas and maintain the "honeymoon period"; and transplanting the pancreas, or at least the islet cells, to reverse the condition once it is fully established. Interventions at diagnosis have been either totally unsuccessful or only minimally successful. There are currently no treatments approved for routine use.

Pancreatic Transplants

The first pancreatic transplants were attempted in the 1960s, and transplants continue to be performed in many centers around the world. The problem with this operation is that the transplanted pancreas is subject to rejection. Recipients must therefore receive high doses of anti-rejection medications, which can have troublesome and significant side-effects, including development of cancer. For people who need a kidney transplant for advanced diabetes-related kidney complications, who will require the use of anti-rejection drugs anyway, transplanting the pancreas at the same time may make good sense. For those well controlled on insulin, with no evidence of kidney complications, transplantation is a less obvious choice. Virtually no transplants have been performed in young people with diabetes.

Islet-cell Transplants

Enormous efforts have been made not only to perfect pancreatic transplantation, but also to isolate the islets and transplant them without the non-insulin-producing parts of the pancreas. However, this technology is still new and has its problems. There is a chronic shortage of pancreases from which to isolate islets, and there are problems with rejection, and technical issues. Even if the technical and rejection problems can be remedied, it is expected that three to five organ donors' pancreases will be needed for each islet transplant recipient. This is a major stumbling block to islet-cell transplants becoming a realistic solution to Type 1 diabetes.

Creating New Islet Cells

The next phase of research involves genetic engineering, in which either animal or non-islet cells are genetically changed to become functioning islet cells. The enormous complexity of islet cell function is being unraveled steadily. This is helping researchers target the genes that must function to make the cells produce and secrete insulin in response to changes in blood glucose levels.

Making Treatment Easier

Although the basic treatment of Type 1 diabetes has changed little over the past 75 years in terms of the need for insulin injections, major advances have been made in a number of areas:

- the variety and purity of insulin preparations, and methods for delivering insulin under the skin, such as insulin pens and pumps
- new and ever-improving methods for monitoring blood glucose and other measures of blood glucose control, such as the hemoglobin A_{1c} test
- the team approach and other approaches to lifestyle management to help prevent psychosocial and long-term physical side-effects.

Insulin

For many years, the only insulins available were relatively

impure preparations of beef and pork insulin. While these were effective in controlling blood glucose levels, they were sometimes associated with side-effects. Over the past 30 years, we have progressed through the development of highly purified pork insulin, to the availability of genetically engineered human insulins, to the recent production of insulin analogs, which are insulins that have been chemically or genetically altered to change their time course of action. Most people with newly diagnosed Type 1 diabetes receive treatment with human insulin, although some centers still prefer the pure pork product. Many are being treated with the superfast-acting insulin analog Lispro, which may be used in place of fast-acting insulin. There are new insulin analogs in various stages of development. Some will be alternatives to fast-acting insulin; others will try to provide the ideal longer-acting basal insulin to which fast-acting insulin is added at mealtime.

Insulin Delivery Systems

Better syringes, finer needles and insulin pens have made insulin injection less painful and more convenient. Smaller and more reliable insulin infusion pumps have also been developed. Pumps don't eliminate the need for a needle or for careful attention to blood sugar control, but they do allow for flexibility in the timing of meals without compromising safety or control. Pumps have not yet met with much enthusiasm from children or teens.

Scientists also continue to work on other methods to administer insulin—for example, by inhalation through the mouth or nose, or through a patch on the skin. This is a highly fertile area of research, in which advances can be expected in the years to come.

Blood Glucose Monitoring

In the late 1970s, urine glucose testing began to be replaced by blood glucose monitoring, a major advance in diabetes management. Over the next 20 years there were significant improvements in monitoring systems, with the development of smaller, more reliable, user-friendly meters with enhanced memory systems, as well as easier-to-use finger-pricking devices.

A major thrust of research continues to be the attempt to develop noninvasive blood glucose testing devices. These would accomplish two things: they would eliminate the need to repeatedly prick the fingers to check blood glucose, and they'd provide the impetus to develop an implantable artificial pancreas, which would detect blood sugar highs or lows, then trigger an insulin pump to infuse the right amount of insulin at the right time. To date, research in this area has been plentiful but a functioning device remains elusive.

Where Do We Go from Here?

Around the world, many researchers remain focused on questions to do with the causes, course and complications of both Type 1 and Type 2 diabetes. They continue to make steady progress, but for many people the pace is too slow. It is clear that there is an ever-increasing need for funding to support research and treatment programs.

Children with diabetes, their families and health care providers, and government and non-governmental organizations that fund diabetes care and research must focus on the challenge at hand: to provide the best available care for people with the disease. It is easy to become disillusioned. Those receiving insulin injections will always hope that a major advance is just around the corner. We need, however, to balance this hope against the reality of where we are in biomedical research, and how much we are likely to advance in the next few years. Following the steps to maintain excellent health now is of critical importance. When advances arrive, children and teens must be well positioned to benefit from them.

Q&A

I keep reading about ancient cures for diabetes and alternative non-drug remedies. How do I know what to believe?
Children with Type 1 diabetes require insulin, which is not a drug. And unfortunately there is no therapy, alternative or otherwise, that eliminates that need. Some people with diabetes find certain nutritional supplements make them feel better. These are probably not harmful, but shouldn't be thought of as part of the diabetes routine. Check with your doctor before taking them.

How can I make sure that I hear about the latest important research in diabetes?
Look to your diabetes team to keep you informed about research that will make a difference to you or your child. It is their responsibility to stay up to date on current treatments and significant advances.

Join the Canadian or American Diabetes Association, and the Juvenile Diabetes Foundation. Membership in all organizations includes a subscription to their publications, which always include the latest research. You may also find useful information on the Internet; see Further Resources, at the end of this book.

We are a family of five. One of our children has diabetes. How can the rest of us find out if we are at high risk for developing diabetes, and be part of a prevention study?

The best way to learn about important clinical research and how you can be involved is to talk to members of your diabetes team. If your child is not receiving ongoing care from a pediatric diabetes team and your doctor is unaware of research opportunities that may interest you, you may want to request referral to a children's center.

Every week I read a story in the paper about some new treatment for diabetes being just around the corner. Yet I have had diabetes for 25 years and my child has had it for 6 years, and we're still having insulin injections, doing more testing and worrying about control. Why do the media report premature research findings?

It's true that a "cure" always seems to be around the corner. There are many reasons why stories often promise more than they deliver. Sometimes, the media misinterpret or sensationalize the information they receive from medical meetings or medical journals. Other times, the researchers themselves give an over-optimistic view of when their research will bear fruit and change the face of diabetes care. Still other times, research that looks promising in its early stages turns out to be not so exciting as the studies continue. Unexpected problems may emerge as treatments are studied over the long haul; initially promising results may not hold up. Read media reports carefully, and ask your health care team or diabetes association about them.

Table of Insulin Types

Type	Made by	Appearance	Timing of action (in hours) Onset	Peak	Duration
Superfast-acting					
Humalog (Lispro)	Eli Lilly	clear	5–10 (min.)	1/2–2	3–4
Short-Acting (fast- or rapid-acting)					
Humulin R (Regular)	Eli Lilly	clear	1/2–1	2–5	6–8
Iletin II Regular	Eli Lilly				
Novolin-Toronto	Novo Nordisk				
Novolin R (Regular)	Novo Nordisk				
Velosulin Human (Regular) Buffered	Novo Nordisk				
Intermediate-Acting					
Humulin N (NPH)	Eli Lilly	cloudy	1–2 1/2	6–15	18–24
Humulin L (Lente)	Eli Lilly				
Iletin II Lente	Eli Lilly				
Iletin II NPH	Eli Lilly				
Novolin N (NPH)	Novo Nordisk				
Novolin L (Lente)	Novo Nordisk				
Long-Acting					
Humulin U (Ultralente)	Lilly	cloudy	4	8–30	28–36
Novolin U (Ultralente)	Novo Nordisk				
Mixtures (numbers show percentage of Regular/NPH)					
Humulin	Lilly	10/90, 20/80, 30/70, 40/60, 50/50			
Novolin	Novo Nordisk	10/90, 20/80, 30/70, 40/60, 50/50			

Note: the timing of action of different insulin preparations is approximate. It may vary from one person to another, from one injection site to another and even from day to day. Absorption of the insulin is affected by skin temperature, physical activity and other factors. The effect of human insulins tends to be somewhat earlier in onset, higher in peak and shorter in duration than the effect of insulins of animal origin. The above table is not a complete list of products available from insulin manufacturers. Please contact your diabetes educator or pharmacist for more information.

Glossary

Albuminuria: presence of protein in the urine. In small amounts, called microalbuminuria, this signals early diabetic nephropathy. Larger amounts, called overt proteinuria or macroproteinuria, suggest advanced nephropathy.

Angiotensin converting enzyme (ACE) inhibitors: medications used to protect the kidney once early nephropathy or high blood pressure has been detected.

Antibodies: proteins produced by the immune system to neutralize foreign proteins (i.e. infectious agents).

Autoimmune disorder: a disease in which the body's immune system mistakenly attacks the body's own tissues. Type 1 diabetes is the result of an autoimmune disorder.

Beta cells: cells in the pancreas that produce insulin.

Diabetic ketoacidosis (DKA): severe dehydration and acidosis that develop when blood sugar is very high and not enough insulin is available to prevent excessive breakdown of fat.

Diabetologist: physician specializing in the care of people with diabetes.

DKA. *See* Diabetic ketoacidosis.

Endocrinologist: physician specializing in the diagnosis and treatment of diabetes and other disorders involving the endocrine (glandular) system.

Glucagon: hormone produced in the pancreas that increases blood sugar by stimulating the liver to release its glucose stores.

Glucose: the form of sugar required by the cells of the body to supply energy.

Glycogen: substance made up of sugar that is stored in the liver and muscle. When cells require sugar for energy, glycogen is changed back into sugar and released into the blood.

Gram: unit of weight in the metric system. There are approximately 30 grams in one ounce.

Hemoglobin A1c (HbA$_{1c}$): blood test used to measure long-term glucose control. Glucose attaches to the hemoglobin in red blood cells in proportion to the average blood sugar level over the life span of the red cell (about three months). Measuring HbA$_{1c}$ levels every three months is the best way to track long-term glucose control.

HLA (histocompatibility locus antigens): "tissue-typing" genes on chromosome six that can control the body's immune response, and provide information on someone's risk of developing diabetes.

Immune system: a complex system that defends the body against viruses, bacteria and other invaders. Sometimes the system malfunctions; *See* Autoimmune disorder.

Insulin: hormone produced in the pancreas which is essential for normal metabolism of glucose.

Insulin receptors: areas of body cells to which insulin attaches to allow glucose to enter the cells.

Islet cell antibodies: antibodies to proteins in the pancreas, often found at the time of diagnosis (or even before diagnosis) of diabetes. Used to detect those at risk of diabetes.

Ketoacidosis. *See* Diabetic ketoacidosis.

Kussmaul breathing: deep, sighing breathing that occurs in diabetic ketoacidosis.

Lipids: fats.

Macrovascular complications: diabetes-related complications that affect the large blood vessels, causing heart attacks, strokes, and poor circulation to the extremities, most commonly the feet.

Macula: area near the center of the eye's retina, responsible for precise vision.

Microalbuminuria. *See* Albuminuria.

Microvascular complications: diabetes-related complications that affect the small blood vessels, such as nephropathy, neuropathy and retinopathy.

Nephropathy: kidney damage that may occur as a result of diabetes.

Neuropathy: nerve damage that may occur as a result of diabetes.

Ophthalmologist: physician who specializes in the diagnosis and treatment of diseases of the eye.

Overt proteinuria. *See* Albuminuria.

Pancreas: organ in the abdomen, behind the stomach, that produces both digestive juices and hormones such as insulin and glucagon.

Retina: center part of the back lining of the eye, which senses light. Its many small blood vessels may become damaged when someone has diabetes for a long time.

Retinopathy: eye damage that may occur as a result of diabetes.

Target range: range of blood sugar within which most results of blood glucose testing should fall.

Thyroid: gland in the lower neck that makes thyroid hormones.

Type 1 diabetes: a form of diabetes that usually begins in childhood and requires treatment with insulin.

Type 2 diabetes: a form of diabetes that usually develops as people age, and can usually be managed through changes in diet and lifestyle.

Further Resources

Organizations

U.S.

The American Diabetes
  Association
1660 Duke Street
Alexandria, VA 22314
(703) 549-1500
Fax: (703) 549-6995
Toll-free: 1-800-342-2383
www.diabetes.org
E-mail: customerservice
  @diabetes.org

The Juvenile Diabetes
  Foundation
120 Wall Street
New York, NY 10005-4001
(212) 785-9500
Toll-free: 1-800-JDF-CURE
www.jdfcure.org
E-mail: info@jdfcure.com
The Canadian Diabetes
  Association

Canada

The Canadian Diabetes
  Association
15 Toronto Street, Suite 800
Toronto, ON M5C 2E3
(416) 363-3373
Fax: (416) 363-3393
Toll-free: 1-800-BANTING
www.diabetes.ca
E-mail: info@cda-nat.org

The Juvenile Diabetes
  Foundation
89 Granton Drive
Richmond Hill, ON L4B 2N5
(905) 889-4171
Toll-free: 1-800-668-0274

Books

American Diabetes Association. *Reflections on Diabetes: 39 Inspirational, Real-life Stories on Living with Diabetes.* Alexandria, VA: American Diabetes Association, 1996.

Betschart, Jean. *It's Time to Learn about Diabetes: A Workbook on Diabetes for Children.* Minneapolis: Chronimed, 1991.

Betschart, Jean, and Susan Tomm. *In Control: A Guide for Teens with Diabetes.* Minneapolis: Chronimed, 1995.

Brackenridge, Betty, and R. Rubin. *Sweet Kids: How to Balance Control and Good Nutrition with Family Peace.* Atlanta: American Diabetes Association, 1996.

Brackenridge, Betty, and Richard Dolinar. *Diabetes 101: A Pure and Simple Guide for People Who Use Insulin.* Minneapolis: Chronimed, 1993.

Chase, Peter. *Understanding Insulin Dependent Diabetes.* Denver: The Guild-CDF, 1995.

Elliott, Joanne. *If Your Child Has Diabetes: An Answer Book for Parents.* New York: Perigee, 1990.

Estridge, Bonnie, and Jo Davies. *Diabetes and Your Teenager.* London: Thursons, with the British Diabetes Association, 1996.

Heegaard, Marge, and Chris Ternand. *When a Family Gets Diabetes.* Minneapolis: DCI, 1990.

Hodgson, Babs. *Courage Unending.* Oakville, ON: My Hope, 1994.

Hollerorth, Hugo J., and Debra Kaplan, with Anna Maria Bertorelli and Joslin Diabetes Center. *Everyone Likes to Eat: How Children Can Eat Most of the Foods They Enjoy and Still Take Care of Their Diabetes.* Minneapolis: Chronimed, 1993.

Kaufman, Miriam. *Easy for You to Say.* Toronto: Key Porter, 1995.

Kaufman, Miriam. *Mothering Teens: Understanding the Adolescent Years.* Toronto: Key Porter, 1997.

Lawlor, M., L. Laffel, B. Anderson and A. Bertorelli. *Caring for Young Children Living with Diabetes—Parent Manual.* Boston: Joslin Diabetes Center, 1996.

McArthur, Robert. *Children Have Diabetes Too: Learning Together as Family.* Calgary: Alberta Children's Hospital, 1986.

MacCracken, Joan. *The Sun and the Rain and the Insulin.* Orono, ME: Tiffen, 1996.

Miller, Judy. *Grilled Cheese at Four O'clock in the Morning.* Alexandria, VA: American Diabetes Association, 1988.

Nemanic, Allison, Gretchen Kauth and Marion J. Franz. *Diabetes Care Made Easy.* Minneapolis: Chronimed, 1992.

Wysocki, Tim. *The Ten Keys to Helping Your Child Grow Up with Diabetes.* Alexandria, VA: American Diabetes Association, 1997.

Cookbooks

Algert, Susan, RD, Barbara Grasse, RD and Annie Durning, RD. *The USCD Healthy Diet for Diabetes: A Comprehensive Nutritional Guide and Cookbook* (University of California at San Diego). Boston: Houghton Mifflin, 1990.

American Diabetes Association. *Month of Meals*. Alexandria, VA: American Diabetes Association, 1990–94.

American Diabetes Association and The American Dietetic Association. *Family Cookbook: Volume IV*. New York: Prentice Hall, 1991.

Bartley, Collen, and John Pateman. *Kid's Choice Cookbook*. Sechelt, BC: Picnics, 1995.

Bowling, Stella. *The Everyday Diabetes Cookbook*. Toronto: Key Porter, 1996.

Canadian Diabetes Association. *Healthy and Hearty Diabetic Cooking*. New York: R.A. Rappaport, 1993.

Cooper, Nancy, RD. *The Joy of Snacks*. Minneapolis: Chronimed, 1991.

Hess, Mary Abbot, RD. *The Art of Cooking for the Diabetic*. Chicago or New York: Contemporary, 1996.

Juliano, Joseph, MD, and Dianne Young. *The Diabetic's Innovative Cookbook: A Positive Approach to Living with Diabetes*. New York: Henry Holt, 1994.

Marks, Betty. *Microwave Diabetes Cookbook*. Chicago: Surrey, 1991.

Registered Dietitians from the University of Alabama at Birmingham. *The Complete Step-by-Step Diabetic Cookbook*. Birmingham, AL: Oxmoor House, 1995.

Webb, Robyn. *Diabetic Meals in 30 Minutes—or Less!* Alexandria, VA: American Diabetes Association, 1996.

Multimedia

"Children with Diabetes," produced by Maxishare Productions, Milwaukee, WI, in association with Children's Hospital Health System of Wisconsin.

"Growing and Living with Diabetes," produced by Cameron McCleery Productions, Toronto, ON, in association with the Canadian Diabetic Association and sponsored by Eli Lilly Canada.

"Living with Diabetes," produced by Maxishare Productions, Milwaukee, WI, in association with the Wisconsin Connection for Children, Hospital of Wisconsin.

"Type 1 Diabetes in Children: A Passport to Knowledge," CD-ROM, produced by Alberta Children's Hospital and the University of Calgary, AB, Canada.

"Understanding Diabetes: Tips for Teachers," produced by Maxishare Productions, Milwaukee, WI, in association with the Wisconsin Connection for Children, Hospital of Wisconsin.

Magazines and the Internet

"Camp Sweeney Diabetes Youth Chat Forum," www.campsweeney.org/yforum.html

"Children with Diabetes," www.childrenwithdiabetes.com

Countdown Canada. Published four times a year by the Diabetes Research Foundation/Juvenile Diabetes Foundation, 89 Granton Drive, Richmond Hill, ON, L4B 2N5.

Diabetes Dialogue. Published four times a year by the Canadian Diabetes Association. Also available at www.diabetes.ca/index.htm

Diabetes Forecast. Published monthly by the American Diabetes Association. Also available (by clicking "Read Our Magazine") at www.org/default.htm

Diabetes Self-Management. Published bi-monthly by R.A. Rappaport Publishing, New York, NY. 1-800-234-0923. Also available at www.diabetes-self-mgmt.com/home.htm/

"Diabetic Data Centre," www.demon.co.uk/diabetic/

"Kids Learn about Diabetes," www.geocities.com/Hotsprings/ 6935/

"Kool Kids Magazine," www.diabetes.com/L2TABLES/L2T 107.htm

KWD Magazine for Kids with Diabetes. Published four times a year; welcomes submissions from readers. Box 22003, RPO Golden Mile, Regina, SK, S4S 7G7, Canada. Fax: (306) 565-2938; e-mail: kwd@sk.sympatico.ca

Index

Numbers in italic indicate boxed text.

ACE inhibitors, 172
Activity. *See* Exercise
Adolescents
  alcohol, 152
  blood sugar target range,
    74
  camps, 133–34
  contraception, 152–53
  coping strategies, 149–50
  diabetes management, 84,
    122–23, 148–51, 160,
    162
  diabetic complications, 165
  driving, 155
  eating disorders, 153–55
  employment, 155–56
  impact of diabetes, 149
  insulin dosages, 47
  normal development, *148*
  smoking, 151
  street drugs, 151–52
  transition to adult health
    care, 185–86, 188–89
  Type 2 diabetes, 17–19
  weight, 94–95
Albuminuria, 168, 172
Alcohol, 152
American Diabetes
  Association, 198
Anger, 119
Angiotensin converting
  enzyme inhibitors, 172
Anorexia nervosa, 153
Anxiety, 119
Arteriosclerosis, 174–75
Autoimmune disorders, 7–8

Banting, Frederick, 34–35
Beans, 56, 68–69
Bedwetting, 14
Best, Charles, 34–35
Biguanides, 19
Bladder infections, 177–78
Blood fats, 166, 168, 175

Blood glucose. *See* Blood
  sugar
Blood pressure, 166, 167,
  175
Blood sugar
  balance, 12–13, 23–25, 30
  and complications, 164,
    166
  effect of exercise, 23,
    27–29, 31–32
  effect of food, 26–27,
    55–58
  effect of insulin, 26
  effect of stress, 29–30
  false low, 105
  and hemoglobin A_{1c}
    levels, 83
  how to check, 76–78
  laboratory tests, 167
  low. *See* Hypoglycemia
  record–keeping, 80–81
  research, 197
  target range, 73, *74*
  when to check, 74–75
Bulimia nervosa, 153

Camps and camping,
  132–34, 188
Canadian Diabetes
  Association, 198
Candy, 68, 136
Carbohydrates, 55–56,

63–65, 70–71
Cataracts, 170
Clinic visits
  assessments, 181–82
  getting the most from,
    184–85
Collip, J.B., 35
Complications
  and blood sugar, 164, *166*
  risk factors, 165–67
  risk reduction, *175*
  screening for, 167–68,
    176–77
  types, 164–65
Contraception, 152–53, 178
Cough syrup, 115

Dairy products, 55, 56
Dehydration, 14, *15*
Denial, 118
Dental checkups, 168
Diabetes Control and
  Complications Trial,
    89–90, 165, *175*
Diabetes mellitus
  causes of Type 1, 7–8,
    191–92
  complications, 163–68
  controlling, 25–26
  defined, 3–4
  diagnosis, 16–17, 18
  feelings about, 118–20

intensive management,
88–90
living with, 121–24
ongoing care, 179–80
preventing progression,
193–95
research, 191–99
Type 2, 17–19, 20
types, 5–6
Diabetic ketoacidosis
causes, 15, 32, 107, 115
preventing, 108
signs and symptoms,
15–16, 107–8, 113
Diagnosis, 16–17, 18
Diaper rash, 16
Diet, *see also* Food
consistency, 65–67
during illness, *110*
eating out, 67
fasting, 70
meal plans, 54–55, 58–65
toddlers, 58–59, 69, 142
Type 2 diabetes, 18–19
vegetarian, 70
Digestive system, 3
DKA. *See* Diabetic
ketoacidosis
Driving, 155
Drugs
adolescent experimenta-
tion, 151–52
for controlling diabetes, 19

for illness, 115
for preventing diabetes,
193
to slow nephropathy, 172

Eating disorders, 153–55
Eggs, 56, 57
Employment, 155–56, 161
Environmental triggers, 7–8,
192
Ethnic susceptibility, 17
Exercise
blood sugar balance, 23,
27–29, 31–32
insulin and food
adjustments, 90–95
Eye
cataracts, 170
checkups, 168, 176–77
retinopathy, 168–70

Family
attitudes and beliefs,
121–22, 127–28
counseling, 182
diabetes management,
83–84, 90, 92–93,
122–24, 157–59
feelings on diagnosis,
118–20
finances, 123–24
genetic research, 193
history, 7, 17, 18, 21

impact of diabetes, 20–21,
    123
strategies for adjustment,
    126–27
Fasting, 70
Fatigue, 13, *15*
Fats
    in blood, 166, 168, 175
    in diet, 56–57, 71
Fear, 119
Feelings, 118–20, 127
Field trips, 131
Finances, 123–24
Fish, 56, *57*
Flu shots, 116
Food, *see also* Diet
    carbohydrate counting,
        63–65
    conversion to energy, 9–12
    effect on blood sugar,
        26–27, 55–58
    exchange system, 60–63,
        70
    fast food, *67*
    gifts, 136
Foot problems, 174, 175
Friends, 21, 125–26
Fruit, *55*

Genetic susceptibility, 7,
    17–18, 21, 192
Glucagon, 102–4, 187
Glucose meters, 76, 77–78,

197
Glucose strips, 76
Growth and development
    adolescents, 148–50
    infants and toddlers,
        139–44
    school–aged children,
        144–47
Guilt, 119–20

Hallowe'en, 68
Health care
    clinic visits, 181–82
    family doctor, 183–84,
        188–89
    importance of follow–up,
        180–81
    research information,
        198–99
    transition to adult care,
        185–86, 188–89
    working with professionals,
        184–85
Hemoglobin A_{1c} testing,
    82–83, 167
Holidays, 68, 134–35,
    187–88
Humalog insulin, 200
Humulin insulins, 200
Hyperglycemia
    causes, 105–6
    defined, 24–25
    signs and symptoms,

106–7
Hyperthyroidism, *183*
Hypoglycemia
  causes, 101
  defined, 24–25
  infants and toddlers, 140
  risk reduction, 104–5, 114
  severe, 101–4
  signs and symptoms,
    97–99
  treatment, 99–100,
    114–15
Hypoglycemic agents, 19
Hypothyroidism, *183*

Iletin insulins, 200
Illness, 108–12, 115–16
Immunological response, 7,
  193–94
Impotence, 174, 178
Infants
  blood sugar target range,
    74
  growth and development,
    139–42
  hypoglycemia, 116, 140
  insulin dosages, 47
  meal planning, 58–59
  signs and symptoms,
    15–16
Infection
  at injection site, 52

kidney or bladder, 177–78
Injections
  air bubbles, 52
  bruising, 51
  equipment, 38–39, 196
  given by others, 38, 49
  given by self, 38, 49–50
  glucagon, 103
  infection, 52
  sites, 42–44
Insulin
  action, 35–36
  buying, 36–37
  discovery of, 34–35
  dosage adjustments,
    83–88, 90–91
  dosages, 47–48
  during illness, 111–12
  equipment, 38–39, 44–50,
    196–97
  injecting, 20, 40–41, 52
  injection sites, 42–44
  lack of, 13–16
  leakage, 50–51
  preparing, 39–40, 41–42,
    49, 51
  reaction. *See* Hypolycemia
  research, 195–96
  role, 8–13, 26
  storing, 37–38
  strength, 36
  too much, 52

types, 35, 200
Insulin shock, 101–4
Insulitis, 194
Insurance policies, 176, 188
Islet–cell creation, 195
Islet–cell transplants,
    194–95

Jet injectors, 45–46
Juvenile Diabetes Foundation,
    198

Ketoacidosis. *See* Diabetic
    ketoacidosis
Ketone tests, 79–80, 86
Kidney failure, 172

Lancing devices, 76–77
Legumes, 56, 68–69
Lente insulin
    action and appearance, 36,
        200
    adjustments, 86
    preparing, 39, 41
    storage, 37
Lispro insulin
    action and appearance, 36,
        200
    adjustments, 86
    preparing, 41
    research, 196

MacLeod, J.J.R., 35
Meals. *See* Diet
Meat, 56, 57
Medical–alert bracelets,
    113–14, 187
Menstruation, 160
Microalbuminuria, 168, 172

Needles, 38–39, 48, 50, 196
Nephropathy, 170, 172,
    177–78
Neuropathy, 173–74
Nicotinamide, 193
Novolin insulins, 200
NPH insulin
    action and appearance, *36*,
        200
    adjustments, 86
    preparing, 39, 41
    storage, 37
Nuts, 56

Obesity, 17, 167, 175
Oils, 57

Pancreas, 3–4, 19
Pancreatic transplants, 194
Pens and cartridges, 44,
    48–49, 196
Pregnancy, 6
Preschoolers. *See* Toddlers
Protein, 56–57

Proteinuria, 172
Pumps, 46–47, 196

Record–keeping, 80–81
Regular insulin
  action and appearance, 36,
    200
  adjustments, 86
  preparing, 41
  storage, 37
Research
  funding, 197
  genetic, 192–93, 195
  into causes, 192–93
  into cures, 193–95, 198,
    199
  into treatment, 195–97
  keeping informed about,
    198–99
Retinopathy, 168–70, 171

Sadness, 118
School, 128–31, 136–37
School–aged children
  coping strategies, 145–47,
    161–62
  impact of diabetes, 145
  normal development,
    144–45
Sexual dysfunction, 174, 178
Siblings, 123, 136
Signs and symptoms

diabetes, 13–16
  healthy infant or toddler,
    141
  hyperglycemia, 106–7
  hypoglycemia, 97–99
  insulin shock, 102
  ketoacidosis, 15–16,
    107–8, 113
  nephropathy, 172
  neuropathy, 173
Smoking, 151, 165, 175, 178
Starches, 55
Stress, 29–30
Sugar (in diet), 55, 68, 71
Sugar substitutes, 71
Sulphonylureas, 19
Support groups, 135
Surgery, 112–13
Symptoms. *See* Signs and
  symptoms
Syringes, 38–39, 196

Tests
  blood sugar, 74–78
  for complications, 167–68,
    176–77
  hemoglobin A$_{1c}$, 82–83
  record–keeping, 80–81
  urinary ketones, 79–80
  urinary sugar, 78–79
Thirst, 14, *15*
Thyroid disease, 168, *183*